Impact of Blood Sugar Levels on Intimate Health

Understanding the Connection Between Glucose Control and Sexual Well-being

Brenda F. Dozier

Gratitude

Dear Reader,

Thank you for deciding to read "Impact of Blood Sugar Levels on Intimate Health: Understanding the Connection Between Glucose Control and Sexual Well-being." The fact that you have chosen to purchase this book is evidence of your dedication to better understanding and improving your health.

My heartfelt appreciation goes out to you for your trust and support. The process of writing this book has been a journey filled with devotion, study, and a genuine desire to share insightful information that has the potential to make a difference in your life. It is not only the validation of this effort that your purchase provides, but it also serves to highlight the significance of addressing such an essential yet frequently neglected component of health.

This book was written to bring awareness to the relationship between blood sugar levels and intimate health. To enhance both your physical and emotional well-being, it is intended to equip you with knowledge and tactics that you can put into practice. A step toward a life that is healthier and more meaningful is the fact that you have an interest in this topic.

It is with sincere gratitude that you have chosen to include this book in your journey. Your commitment to learning and improving is inspiring, and it fuels the passion for continued exploration and sharing of knowledge.

With heartfelt gratitude,

[Brenda F. Dozier]

Table of Contents

Introduction

It is of the utmost importance that we have a solid awareness of our well-being in our fast-paced society, where physical health is frequently sacrificed to achieve success and maximize convenience. Maintaining healthy blood sugar levels stands out among the various health concerns we confront because of its substantial and far-reaching influence on those affected by it. Many people may be unaware of the close relationship that exists between the regulation of blood sugar and our sexual health. This is a connection that, if disregarded, can result in substantial and life-altering effects.

In the book "Impact of Blood Sugar Levels on Intimate Health: Understanding the Connection Between Glucose Control and Sexual Well-Being", the author provides a complete guide intended to shine a light on this essential part of health that is sometimes disregarded. Consider the possibility of recovering command of your body and mind, experiencing an increase in your energy levels, and restoring your vitality in the context of your intimate relationships. When you take the time to regulate your blood sugar levels intelligently, this is not only a fantasy but rather a tangible reality that you can achieve.

Have you ever pondered the reasoning behind why, despite your best efforts, your personal life seems to be stressful or lacking in satisfaction? The explanation could lie in the invisible variations of your blood sugar.

Elevated glucose levels do not just offer a danger for diabetes—they cascade into numerous health issues, including those that directly influence sexual desire, performance, and satisfaction. This may result in difficulties with erectile dysfunction for men, while women may notice a decline in their desire or physical pain. These problems, which are frequently kept hidden from view, have the potential to undermine the foundation of our most intimate relationships and to have an effect on our quality of life in general.

To provide you with knowledge and strategies that you may put into practice, this book was written. It bridges the gap between medical knowledge and everyday application, taking you on a journey towards greater health and more rewarding intimate relationships. You'll discover how simple modifications in nutrition, exercise, and lifestyle can stabilize your blood sugar levels and, in turn, revive your sexual health. By understanding the hormonal and physiological underpinnings, you will obtain a new perspective on the necessity of glucose regulation.

In these pages, you'll also find inspiring stories from individuals and case studies that highlight the real-world benefits of maintaining balanced blood sugar levels. These accounts not only offer optimism but also highlight the concrete gains in sexual health and overall well-being that come with attentive glucose management. Through these stories, you will learn that you are not alone in your challenges and that there is a road ahead to a healthier, happier life.

As we look to the future, we study the newest research and technology developments, offering you a peek at the technologies that are defining the future of diabetes treatment and sexual health.

Ultimately, Impact of Blood Sugar Levels on Intimate Health is more than simply a book; it's a call to action to take control of your health and your life, to understand the connections inside your body, and to cultivate a deeper, more meaningful intimate relationship. This is your guide to not just surviving but thriving, with the knowledge that every small step you take towards better blood sugar management is a step towards a healthier, happier self.

Let this book be your companion as you traverse the path to better health and intimacy. Embrace the power of information, and let it transform your life. Together, we can disclose the secrets of how blood sugar levels affect intimate health, unleashing the possibility of a vibrant and full existence.

Purpose of the Book

The primary purpose of this book is to focus attention on the often-overlooked connection between blood sugar levels and intimate health. By completely examining how glucose control influences sexual well-being, this book strives to empower readers with the knowledge and techniques needed to better both their physical health and romantic relationships. In a world where diabetes and prediabetes are increasingly frequent, understanding the larger consequences of blood sugar management is vital. This book is meant for people impacted by blood sugar disorders, healthcare professionals, and anybody interested in health and wellness.

This book goes beyond the basic advice commonly found in health guidelines, presenting a full investigation of the physiological, psychological, and emotional elements of sexual health as they relate to blood sugar levels. It tries to fill a gap in existing literature by addressing a topic that is crucial yet infrequently explored. By providing concrete insights and practical solutions, this book inspires readers to take control of their health, improve their quality of life, and enrich their intimate relationships.

Explaining the Significance of Understanding Blood Sugar Levels and Their Impact on Intimate Health

Blood sugar, or glucose, is a serious energy source for the body's cells. Proper management of blood sugar levels is vital for maintaining general health and preventing chronic illnesses such as diabetes. However, the significance of blood sugar management extends beyond preventing diabetes-related problems. It also plays a critical role in maintaining sexual health and intimate relationships, areas that are strongly influenced by physical well-being.

High or low blood sugar levels can contribute to different health issues, including those that harm interpersonal health. For instance, hyperglycemia (high blood sugar) can cause damage to blood vessels and neurons, leading to issues such as erectile dysfunction in males and decreased libido in women. Hypoglycemia (low blood sugar), on the other hand, can result in weariness, irritation, and anxiety, all of which can significantly impair romantic relationships and sexual performance.

Understanding the association between blood sugar levels and intimate health encourages individuals to appreciate the need to keep stable glucose levels. It highlights the interdependence of physical health and sexual well-being, underscoring the necessity for a holistic approach to health management. By understanding these signs and symptoms of blood sugar abnormalities and their possible impact on intimate health, individuals may take proactive actions to address these concerns and improve their overall quality of life.

Why It Matters: Highlighting the Impact of Glucose Control on Overall Health and Quality of Life

The regulation of blood sugar levels is crucial for overall health and well-being. Poor glucose regulation can lead to several health concerns, ranging from minor to severe. Chronic high blood sugar levels, for example, can result in consequences such as cardiovascular disease, kidney damage, and nerve damage. These disorders not only impair physical health but also have a dramatic impact on quality of life, reducing one's capacity to engage in everyday activities and lead a happy existence.

In terms of sexual health, glucose regulation is similarly crucial. Sexual dysfunctions such as erectile dysfunction in males and decreased libido in women are frequent difficulties connected with poor blood sugar management. These difficulties can lead to substantial emotional and psychological suffering, hurting self-esteem, confidence, and intimate relationships. The pressure on romantic relationships can further worsen stress and anxiety, producing a vicious cycle that severely undermines general well-being.

Effective glucose control can prevent these issues, ensuring better physical health and enhancing quality of life. By maintaining stable blood sugar levels, individuals can lower the chance of acquiring chronic illnesses and improve their sexual health. This, in turn, leads to healthier intimate connections and a more fulfilling life. The capacity to manage blood sugar successfully empowers individuals to take charge of their health, enhancing both physical and mental well-being.

Overview of the Relationship Between Glucose Control and Sexual Well-being

The association between glucose regulation and sexual well-being is complicated, comprising different physiological, psychological, and emotional aspects. Blood sugar levels influence the body's ability to function optimally, affecting everything from energy levels to hormone balance. These elements are vital for maintaining sexual health and performance.

For men, glucose regulation is closely linked to erectile function. High blood sugar levels can damage blood vessels and nerves, limiting blood flow to the penis and resulting in erectile dysfunction. Additionally, improper glucose control can influence testosterone levels, lowering libido and sexual desire. For women, blood sugar abnormalities can lead to vaginal dryness, decreased libido, and irregular menstrual cycles, all of which can severely impair sexual health.

The psychological and emotional components of glucose control are as important. Blood sugar changes can contribute to mood swings, anxiety, and sadness, all of which can influence sexual desire and performance.

Chronic stress and worry connected to regulating blood sugar levels can further strain romantic relationships, lowering overall satisfaction and connection with a partner.

Maintaining stable blood sugar levels maintains hormonal balance, appropriate blood flow, and nerve activity, all of which are crucial for sexual health. It also helps to relieve tension and anxiety, providing a happy emotional state that is conducive to healthy intimate relationships. By recognizing the intricate relationship between glucose control and sexual well-being, individuals can make proactive efforts to improve their health and enhance their intimate lives.

Thesis Statement: Maintaining Healthy Blood Sugar Levels is Crucial for Optimal Sexual Health and Intimate Relationships

Maintaining balanced blood sugar levels is vital for optimal sexual health and romantic relationships. Proper glucose regulation not only prevents chronic health issues but also promotes the physiological, psychological, and emotional components required for sexual well-being. By knowing and managing blood sugar levels, individuals can improve their overall health, boost their sexual health, and build happier, more meaningful romantic relationships.

Effective blood sugar management begins with a full grasp of how glucose levels affect the body. This includes detecting the signs and symptoms of blood sugar abnormalities and understanding their potential impact on sexual health. By adopting a holistic approach to health management that includes a balanced diet, regular exercise, and stress management techniques, individuals can maintain stable blood sugar levels and enhance overall well-being.

A balanced diet is crucial to blood sugar regulation. Consuming nutrient-rich foods that maintain steady glucose levels helps minimize blood sugar spikes and crashes. Food's high in fiber, healthy fats, and lean proteins are particularly advantageous, as they induce satiety and regulate glucose absorption. Avoiding sugary meals and refined carbohydrates also helps maintain stable blood sugar levels, minimizing the risk of issues that can compromise sexual health.

Regular exercise is another main component of blood sugar regulation. Physical activity helps manage glucose levels by enhancing insulin sensitivity and promoting glucose absorption by muscles. This not only helps general health but also enhances sexual health by facilitating optimal blood flow and hormone balance. Engaging in regular physical activity, such as aerobic exercise and strength training, helps maintain healthy blood sugar levels and supports good sexual performance.

Stress management techniques are also helpful for maintaining stable blood sugar levels. Chronic stress can lead to higher cortisol levels, which can significantly affect glucose control and general health. Practices such as mindfulness meditation, yoga, and deep breathing exercises can help reduce stress and increase emotional well-being. By handling stress efficiently, individuals can improve their blood sugar control and boost their sexual health.

Healthcare practitioners play a critical role in aiding people with blood sugar management. Regular check-ups and monitoring of blood sugar levels can identify potential concerns early and provide opportunities for action. Open communication with healthcare practitioners regarding sexual health concerns is vital, as it allows for a comprehensive approach to health management. By working together with healthcare specialists, individuals can establish tailored programs to maintain appropriate blood sugar levels and improve their sexual health.

The relationship between blood sugar control and sexual health highlights the necessity of a holistic approach to health management. By understanding the connection between glucose levels and sexual well-being, individuals can make proactive efforts to improve their general health and enrich their romantic relationships.

This book attempts to provide the knowledge and resources needed to handle these issues, empowering readers to take charge of their health and experience a satisfying, vibrant life.

Chapter 1

Understanding Blood Sugar and Its Regulation

Blood sugar, commonly known as blood glucose, is a crucial component of our body's metabolic functions. It serves as the major source of energy for our cells, fueling everything from basic physiological operations to complicated cerebral tasks. The management of blood sugar levels is essential for maintaining overall health and preventing several chronic disorders, including diabetes. This chapter tries to provide a comprehensive explanation of what blood sugar is, how it is regulated in the body, and the ramifications of its dysregulation, specifically addressing insulin resistance and its impact on personal health.

What is blood sugar?

Blood sugar refers to the concentration of glucose present in the bloodstream. Glucose is a simple sugar and an essential carbohydrate that the body gets from the meals we ingest. It is the primary source of energy for our cells, tissues, and organs, particularly the brain, which relies largely on glucose to function correctly.

Definition and Explanation of Blood Glucose

Glucose enters the bloodstream during the digestive process, where carbs from food are broken down. The digestion of carbohydrates starts in the mouth with the action of salivary amylase and continues in the small intestine, where enzymes further break down complex carbs into glucose. Once absorbed through the intestinal walls, glucose enters the bloodstream, ready to be delivered to cells for energy production.

The body methodically manages blood glucose levels to ensure they remain within a restricted range. This management is crucial because both high and low blood sugar levels can have detrimental consequences on health. The typical fasting blood glucose level for a non-diabetic person from the ranges between 70 and 99 mg/dL. After meals, blood glucose levels can rise initially, but they normally fall to the fasting range within a few hours.

Two important hormones, insulin, and glucagon, performant dynamic roles in maintaining blood glucose homeostasis. Insulin, produced by the beta cells of the pancreas, stimulates the uptake of glucose by cells, allowing it to be utilized for energy or stored as glycogen in the liver and muscles. Glucagon, produced by the alpha cells of the pancreas, has the opposite effect; it increases the release of glucose from glycogen stores in the liver when blood sugar levels dip too low.

Insulin Resistance: How Persistent High Blood Sugar Leads to Insulin Resistance and Its Implications for Intimate Health

Insulin resistance is a state where the body's cells become less receptive to the hormone insulin. This illness commonly occurs after lengthy periods of increased blood sugar levels, typically owing to poor food, lack of exercise, and other lifestyle issues. When insulin resistance emerges, the body needs to create more insulin to maintain normal blood glucose levels, leading to hyperinsulinemia (excess levels of insulin in the blood).

The development of insulin resistance is a slow process that might eventually lead to type 2 diabetes if not treated effectively. In insulin resistance, the cells in the muscles, fat, and liver start rejecting or refusing the signal from insulin to take in glucose from the bloodstream. As a result, glucose levels remain high, leading the pancreas to release even more insulin in an attempt to lower blood sugar levels.

Persistently elevated blood sugar and insulin resistance have several major implications for intimate health. One of the key areas affected is sexual health, where both men and women can face numerous difficulties.

Implications for Men's Intimate Health

In men, insulin resistance and excessive blood sugar levels can lead to erectile dysfunction (ED). Erectile function depends on a healthy vascular system and proper blood flow to the penile tissue. Chronic high blood sugar levels might harm the blood vessels and nerves that are needed to achieves and sustains an erection. This injury is typically referred to as diabetic neuropathy when it happens in the context of diabetes.

Additionally, insulin resistance is commonly related to reduced testosterone levels in men, a condition known as hypogonadism. Testosterone is vital for maintaining libido and general sexual health. Low amounts of this hormone can contribute to lower sexual desire, energy levels, and mood, further exacerbating the difficulty of sustaining a good personal connection.

Implications for Women's Intimate Health

Women also experience substantial intimate health concerns due to insulin resistance and excessive blood sugar levels. One common condition is vaginal dryness, which can make sexual intercourse uncomfortable or painful. This disorder often originates from hormonal abnormalities induced by insulin resistance, which can affect the normal production of estrogen and other sex hormones.

Insulin resistance can also lead to polycystic ovary syndrome (PCOS), a disorder characterized by irregular menstrual periods, ovarian cysts, and increased levels of male hormones. Women with PCOS often have diminished fertility, acne, and hirsutism (excessive hair growth), which can damage their self-esteem and intimate relationships.

Moreover, insulin resistance can worsen weight gain, particularly in the abdominal region. Excess body weight, especially around the midsection, is associated with increased production of inflammatory cytokines and decreased synthesis of sex hormone-binding globulin (SHBG), which can further disturb hormonal balance and sexual health.

The Broader Impact of Insulin Resistance on Health

Beyond its specific consequences on intimate health, insulin resistance has far-reaching implications for overall health. It is a major risk factor for the development of metabolic syndrome, a cluster of disorders that includes hypertension, dyslipidemia (abnormal cholesterol levels), and abdominal obesity. Metabolic syndrome dramatically raises the risk of cardiovascular disease, stroke, and type 2 diabetes.

Insulin resistance also promotes systemic inflammation, which can damage blood vessels and organs throughout the body. Chronic inflammation is a critical element in the development of atherosclerosis (the buildup of fatty deposits in the arteries), leading to heart attacks and strokes. This systemic impact underlines the need to regulate blood sugar levels to prevent long-term health consequences.

The Role of Insulin in Regulating Blood Sugar Levels

Insulin is a vital hormone in the body, largely responsible for controlling blood sugar (glucose) levels. Produced by the beta cells of the pancreas, insulin stimulates the uptake of glucose by cells, allowing it to be used for energy or stored for future use. Understanding the role of insulin is vital for appreciating how blood sugar levels are maintained and what occurs when this process is interrupted.

When we eat carbs, they are broken down into glucose, which enters the bloodstream. The rise in blood glucose levels prompts the pancreas to release insulin. Insulin operates like a key, opening cells so that glucose may enter and be consumed for energy. Without insulin, or if the body grows resistant to its actions, glucose continues in the bloodstream, resulting in increased blood sugar levels.

Insulin has various key functions, including:

Facilitating Glucose Uptake: Insulin attaches to receptors on cell surfaces, notably in muscle and fat regions, signaling these cells to absorb glucose from the bloodstream.

Regulating Glycogen Storage: In the liver, insulin promotes the conversion of excess glucose into glycogen for storage. When blood sugar levels decline, glycogen can be broken down back into glucose to sustain energy levels.

Inhibiting Gluconeogenesis: Insulin slows the creation of glucose from non-carbohydrate sources in the liver, a process known as gluconeogenesis. This helps avoid excessive glucose release into the bloodstream.

Promoting Lipogenesis: Insulin stimulates the storage of excess glucose as fat in adipose tissue. While this is a valuable mechanism for energy storage, excessive insulin activity can lead to weight gain.

When the body develops insulin resistance, the cells do not respond efficiently to the hormone, resulting in higher blood glucose levels. The pancreas adjusts by making more insulin, but over time, this can lead to beta cell exhaustion and type 2 diabetes. Insulin resistance is commonly connected with obesity, physical inactivity, and poor diet, making lifestyle changes vital for prevention and management.

How Blood Sugar Levels Are Measured

Accurate measurement of blood sugar levels is vital for identifying and managing illnesses like diabetes. Blood sugar levels can be monitored using numerous methods, each offering valuable information regarding glucose regulation over different times. Understanding these strategies helps individuals and healthcare providers make educated decisions regarding treatment and lifestyle improvements.

Methods of Blood Sugar Testing

Fasting Glucose Test

The fasting glucose test measures blood sugar levels after an individual has no eat for at least 8 hours. It is commonly conducted in the morning, before breakfast. This test gives a glimpse of how the body maintains blood sugar levels without the influence of recent food intake.

Procedure: A blood sample is obtained from a vein in the arm, and the glucose concentration is measured.

Normal Range: A normal fasting blood glucose level is normally between 70 and 99 mg/dL.

Prediabetes: Levels between 100 and 125 mg/dL suggest prediabetes, a condition where blood sugar levels are higher than usual but not yet high enough for a diabetes diagnosis.

Diabetes: A fasting blood glucose level of 126 mg/dL or above on two independent tests usually indicates diabetes.

The fasting glucose test is a good approach for identifying diabetes and prediabetes. It is typically used in conjunction with other tests to confirm a diagnosis and assess the success of diabetes management measures.

A1C Test

The A1C test, commonly known as the hemoglobin A1C or HbA1c test, measures the average blood sugar levels over the last two to three months. It shows the percentage of hemoglobin, the oxygen-carrying protein in red blood cells, that is coated with glucose.

Procedure: A blood sample is obtained from a vein in the arm, and the percentage of glycated hemoglobin is measured.

Normal Range: An A1C level below 5.7% is measured normal.

Prediabetes: An A1C reading between 5.7% and 6.4% suggests prediabetes.

Diabetes: An A1C score of 6.5% or above on two separate tests suggests diabetes.

The A1C test is particularly beneficial because it does not require fasting and provides a long-term view of blood sugar control. It is often used to assess the success of diabetes therapy and to make modifications to medication and lifestyle treatments.

Glucose Tolerance Test (GTT)

The glucose tolerance test examines the body's capacity to control glucose over a period of time. It is typically used to diagnose gestational diabetes during pregnancy but can also be used to diagnose type 2 diabetes and prediabetes.

Procedure: The test begins with a fasting blood glucose measurement. The user then takes a sweet drink with a certain amount of glucose (typically 75 grams). Blood sugar levels are monitored at regular intervals, often at one, two, and sometimes three hours after eating the drink.

Normal Range: For the two-hour test, a blood sugar level below 140 mg/dL is considered normal.

Prediabetes: A two-hour blood sugar level between 140 and 199 mg/dL suggests prediabetes.

Diabetes: A two-hour blood sugar level of 200 mg/dL or greater suggests diabetes.

The glucose tolerance test provides information about how fast glucose is eliminated from the bloodstream and how well the body responds to an inflow of sugar. It is a comprehensive test that can detect anomalies in glucose metabolism that other tests might overlook.

Continuous Glucose Monitoring (CGM)

Continuous glucose monitoring (CGM) systems provide real-time data on blood sugar levels throughout the day and night. These gadgets are particularly useful for those with diabetes who need to closely monitor their glucose levels to manage their disease successfully.

Procedure: A tiny sensor is implanted beneath the skin, generally on the belly or arm. The sensor monitors glucose levels in the interstitial fluid (the fluid surrounding the cells) and sends the data to a receiver or smartphone.

Benefits: CGM systems give continuous data, enabling the detection of patterns and trends in blood sugar levels. They can inform users of high or low glucose levels, helping to avert severe episodes of hyperglycemia or hypoglycemia.

Limitations: While CGM systems offer valuable insights, they require regular calibration with traditional blood glucose monitors and may not be as reliable as lab-based examinations.

CGM systems are becoming increasingly popular for treating diabetes, providing a thorough picture of blood sugar variations and helping to fine-tune treatment strategies.

Importance of Regular Blood Sugar Testing

Regular blood sugar testing is vital for treating diabetes and preventing complications. For people with diabetes, frequent monitoring helps ensure that blood sugar levels remain within target ranges, minimizing the risk of consequences such as cardiovascular disease, neuropathy, and kidney damage. For those at risk of diabetes, routine testing can reveal blood sugar problems early, allowing for prompt actions to avoid the progression of diabetes.

Interpreting Blood Sugar Levels

Understanding the results of blood sugar tests is vital for optimal diabetic control. Each test provides particular information that can influence treatment decisions:

Fasting Glucose Test: Indicates how well the body maintains blood sugar levels in the absence of food. High levels signal poor glucose management and probable insulin resistance.

A1C Test: Giving an average blood sugar level over the past two to three months, showing long-term glucose control. Higher levels signal the need for modifications in diet, exercise, or medication.

Glucose Tolerance Test: The test assesses the body's response to a glucose challenge, offering information into how rapidly glucose is removed from the bloodstream. Abnormal results indicate impaired glucose tolerance or diabetes.

Continuous Glucose Monitoring: Offers real-time data on blood sugar variations, helping to spot patterns and adapt treatment accordingly.

Healthcare providers utilize these tests in combination to gain a thorough picture of an individual's glucose metabolism and to customize treatment strategies accordingly.

Factors Affecting Blood Sugar Levels

Several factors can alter blood sugar levels, making regular testing and monitoring essential:

Diet: Carbohydrate intake has a substantial impact on blood sugar levels. Consuming high-glycemic foods, which are rapidly digested and absorbed, which can make rises in blood sugar levels. A balanced diet with low-glycemic foods helps maintain steady glucose levels.

Physical Activity: Exercise raises insulin sensitivity and promotes glucose uptake by muscles, reducing blood sugar levels. Regular physical activity is vital for treating diabetes and boosting overall health.

Drugs: Certain drugs, such as insulin and oral hypoglycemics, are used to regulate blood sugar levels. Adjustments in medication dosage may be necessary based on blood sugar test results.

Stress: Stress can alter blood sugar levels by increasing the production of hormones such as cortisol, which can boost blood sugar levels. Managing stress through approaches such as meditation, exercise, and enough sleep is important for blood sugar control.

Illness: Illness and infections can cause blood sugar levels to vary, making continuous monitoring vital during periods of illness.

Normal vs. Abnormal Blood Sugar Levels

Understanding the distinction between normal and abnormal blood sugar levels is vital for maintaining general health and preventing chronic illnesses such as diabetes. Blood sugar, or glucose, is the principal energy source for the body's cells. It is crucial to keep blood sugar levels within a specified range to ensure that the body works efficiently. Abnormal levels can lead to major health complications, both in the near term and over the long term. This chapter presents a comprehensive overview of what constitutes normal blood sugar levels, the ramifications of deviations from these levels, and the conditions of hyperglycemia and hypoglycemia.

Range of Normal Blood Sugar Levels

Normal blood sugar levels fluctuate depending on the time of day, dietary intake, and individual health conditions. Generally, there are established ranges that medical experts use to determine whether blood sugar levels are within a safe range.

Fasting Blood Sugar Levels

Fasting blood sugar levels are assessed when an individual has not eaten for at least eight hours, often taken in the morning before breakfast. This metric helps to examine how well the body maintains blood sugar levels without the effects of recent food intake.

Normal Range: For a healthy individual, fasting blood sugar levels normally range from 70 to 99 mg/dL (milligrams per deciliter).

Prediabetes: A fasting blood sugar level between 100 and 125 mg/dL is indicative of prediabetes, a disease where blood sugar levels are raised but not high enough to be categorized as diabetes.

Diabetes: A fasting blood sugar level of 126 mg/dL or above on two different occasions usually indicates diabetes.

Postprandial Blood Sugar Levels

Postprandial blood sugar levels are assessed two hours after eating. This measurement aids to understand how the body handles glucose after a meal.

Normal Range: For non-diabetic individuals, postprandial blood sugar levels are normally less than 140 mg/dL two hours after eating.

Prediabetes: Levels between 140 and 199 mg/dL suggest decreased glucose tolerance or prediabetes.

Diabetes: A reading of 200 mg/dL or greater two hours after eating is indicative of diabetes.

A1C Levels

The A1C test, commonly known as the hemoglobin A1C or HbA1c test, offers an average of blood sugar levels over the last two to three months. This test examines the percentage of hemoglobin that is glycated, or coated with sugar.

Normal Range: An A1C level below 5.7% is measured normal.

Prediabetes: An A1C reading between 5.7% and 6.4% suggests prediabetes.

Diabetes: An A1C score of 6.5% or above on two independent tests is indicative of diabetes.

Definitions and Implications of Hyperglycemia and Hypoglycemia

Hyperglycemia and hypoglycemia describe conditions with unusually high and low blood sugar levels, respectively. Both disorders have substantial health implications and require cautious management to avoid serious complications.

Hyperglycemia

Hyperglycemia refers to increased blood sugar levels. It occurs when the body does not create enough insulin or when the cells become resistant to insulin, preventing glucose from being properly absorbed from the bloodstream.

Definition: Hyperglycemia is commonly characterized as blood sugar levels above 130 mg/dL before a meal or above 180 mg/dL two hours after a meal.

Causes: Common causes of hyperglycemia include diabetes, high carbohydrate intake, physical inactivity, stress, illness, and some drugs.

Symptoms: Symptoms of hyperglycemia includes frequent urination, increased thirst, impaired vision, lethargy, and headaches. Severe hyperglycemia can lead to more significant symptoms such as disorientation, shortness of breath, and fruity-smelling breath.

Implications of Hyperglycemia

Chronic hyperglycemia can have significant health repercussions, particularly for people with diabetes. Long-term increased blood sugar levels can damage blood vessels and neurons, leading to issues such as:

Cardiovascular Disease: Persistent high blood sugar can damage the blood vessels, increasing the risk of heart disease, stroke, and hypertension.

Neuropathy: High blood sugar can damage nerves, particularly in the legs and feet, leading to numbness, discomfort, and, in extreme cases, infection and amputation.

Retinopathy: Damage to the blood vessels in the retina can lead to vision issues and possibly blindness.

Renal Damage: High blood sugar levels can damage the kidneys' filtering function, leading to renal disease and, eventually, kidney failure.

Poor Wound Healing: Elevated blood sugar levels can hinder the body's capacity to heal wounds, increasing the risk of infections.

Managing Hyperglycemia

Effective therapy for hyperglycemia entails a combination of lifestyle changes and, where necessary, medication. Strategies include:

Dietary Changes: Adopting a balanced diet low in refined carbohydrates and high in fiber will help manage blood sugar levels.

Regular Exercise: Physical activity promotes insulin sensitivity and helps lower blood sugar levels.

Medication: In some circumstances, oral medicines or insulin therapy may be essential to maintain blood sugar levels within a normal range.

Monitoring: Regular monitoring of blood sugar levels helps individuals make informed decisions regarding their nutrition, activity, and medication.

Hypoglycemia

Hypoglycemia refers to abnormally low blood sugar levels. It occurs when there is too much insulin in the bloodstream relative to the amount of glucose, leading to a quick decline in blood sugar levels.

Definition: Hypoglycemia is generally characterized as blood sugar levels below 70 mg/dL.

Causes: Common causes include excessive insulin administration, some diabetes medicines, prolonged fasting, heavy alcohol usage, and physical activity.

Symptoms: Symptoms of hypoglycemia can include shakiness, sweating, disorientation, irritability, rapid heartbeat, and dizziness. Severe hypoglycemia can lead to seizures, loss of consciousness, and even death if not properly treated.

Implications of Hypoglycemia

Hypoglycemia can have immediate and even life-threatening effects, particularly for patients with diabetes who are on insulin therapy or other glucose-lowering drugs. Repeated episodes of hypoglycemia can also develop into hypoglycemia unawareness, where the individual no longer perceives early warning indicators, increasing the likelihood of severe episodes.

Cognitive Impairment: Low blood sugar can affect brain function, leading to confusion, trouble concentrating, and poor coordination.

Accidents and Injuries: Severe hypoglycemia can cause fainting or seizures, increasing the risk of accidents and injuries.

Cardiovascular Stress: Hypoglycemia can produce a rapid increase in heart rate and blood pressure, potentially initiating cardiovascular events in sensitive individuals.

Managing Hypoglycemia

Effective therapy for hypoglycemia entails recognizing the early signs and taking fast steps to boost blood sugar levels. Strategies include:

Immediate Treatment: Consuming fast-acting carbs such as glucose tablets, fruit juice, or candies will swiftly raise blood sugar levels.

Monitoring: Regular blood sugar monitoring helps uncover tendencies that may lead to hypoglycemia, allowing for prompt adjustments in food, activity, and medication.

Medication Adjustment: For patients with diabetes, adjusting the amount of insulin or other glucose-lowering drugs can help prevent episodes of hypoglycemia.

Dietary Management: Eating frequent meals and snacks that include complex carbs, protein, and healthy fats will help maintain stable blood sugar levels.

Maintaining blood sugar levels within a normal range is vital for overall health and well-being. Understanding the differences between normal and abnormal blood sugar levels, as well as the situations of hyperglycemia and hypoglycemia, is critical for preventing and managing diabetes and its complications. Regular monitoring, lifestyle adjustments, and appropriate medication interventions are critical measures for achieving optimal blood sugar management and minimizing the risk of major health concerns. By keeping informed and proactive, individuals can take control of their blood sugar levels and improve their quality of life.

Weight gain, kidney damage and sexual health are harmful effects of excess sugar

Excessive sugar intake has far-reaching repercussions on general health, contributing considerably to weight gain, renal damage, and sexual health difficulties. Understanding these consequences can drive individuals to adopt healthier dietary habits and lifestyle choices.

Weight Gain

One of the most apparent and visible outcomes of excessive sugar consumption is weight gain. Sugar, mostly in the form of fructose, contributes to the development of obesity in numerous ways:

Caloric Excess: Sugary foods and beverages are high in calories but low in nutritional value. Consuming these calorie-dense foods leads to an energy imbalance, where the intake exceeds the expenditure, resulting in weight gain. Unlike complex carbs, which are digested slowly and provide a consistent supply of energy, simple sugars are swiftly taken into the bloodstream, resulting in abrupt spikes and subsequent drops in blood sugar levels. This quick variation often causes hunger and desires, driving further caloric intake.

Insulin Resistance: Excess sugar intake, particularly from fructose, can contribute to insulin resistance. Insulin is a hormone that controls blood sugar levels by facilitating the uptake of glucose into cells for energy production or storage. When cells become resistant to insulin, the body adapts by manufacturing more insulin, resulting in higher insulin levels (hyperinsulinemia). Elevated insulin levels encourage fat storage, especially in the abdominal area, and make it difficult to reduce weight. This insulin resistance is a fundamental aspect of metabolic syndrome, a collection of diseases that increase the risk of heart disease, stroke, and diabetes.

Leptin Resistance: Leptin is a hormone generated by fat cells that instructs the brain to manage hunger and energy balance. High sugar intake can contribute to leptin resistance when the brain does not respond to leptin signals adequately. This resistance results in chronic sensations of hunger and lower energy expenditure, further promoting weight gain. The pattern of overeating and weight gain exacerbates leptin resistance, producing a vicious spiral that is hard to break.

Addictive tendencies: Sugar contains addictive tendencies that can lead to overeating. It affects the brain's reward system, releasing dopamine, a chemical associated with pleasure and reward. This activation provides a sense of euphoria, comparable to addictive medications, which can lead to habitual consumption and reliance. Over time, the brain demands bigger amounts of sugar to generate the same pleasurable effects, leading to increasing caloric consumption and weight gain.

Metabolic Consequences: Excess sugar intake can alter normal metabolic functions. High levels of sugar in the diet can affect the gut microbiota, the population of microorganisms living in the digestive tract, leading to dysbiosis (an imbalance in the gut flora). This imbalance can contribute to metabolic problems, inflammation, and weight gain. Additionally, fructose metabolism in the liver produces uric acid, which can impede insulin signaling and contribute to insulin resistance and weight gain.

Kidney Damage

The kidneys perform a key function in filtering waste items from the blood, controlling fluid and electrolyte balance, and maintaining overall homeostasis. Excessive sugar intake can have adverse consequences on renal function:

Hyperglycemia: Chronic high blood sugar levels, usually found in persons with uncontrolled diabetes, can damage the blood vessels in the kidneys. This disorder, known as diabetic nephropathy, is a significant cause of chronic kidney disease (CKD). Hyperglycemia increases the pressure within the glomeruli (the filtering units of the kidneys), causing them to become damaged and less effective at filtering waste. Over time, this damage can lead to proteinuria (the presence of protein in urine), a symptom of renal impairment.

Hypertension: High sugar intake, particularly from sugary beverages, is related to an increased risk of hypertension (high blood pressure). Hypertension is a key risk factor for renal disease, as it puts additional strain on the blood arteries in the kidneys, leading to damage and impaired kidney function. The combination of hypertension and hyperglycemia can speed the progression of renal disease.

Oxidative Stress: Excess sugar consumption can promote oxidative stress, a condition characterized by an imbalance between the creation of free radicals and the body's ability to neutralize them with antioxidants. Oxidative stress can damage kidney cells and tissues, affecting their function. High sugar intake also stimulates the creation of advanced glycation end products (AGEs), which are toxic molecules that form when proteins or lipids interact with sugar in the bloodstream. AGEs lead to oxidative stress and inflammation, further harming the kidneys.

Increased Risk of Kidney Stones: Excessive sugar consumption, particularly from fructose, can raise the risk of kidney stones. Fructose increases urine excretion of calcium, oxalate, and uric acid, which are significant components of kidney stones. High sugar intake can also lead to dehydration, another risk factor for kidney stone formation. Proper hydration is crucial for diluting urine and preventing the crystallization of stone-forming chemicals.

Sexual Health

Sexual health is a vital element of general well-being, and high sugar intake can have major negative implications on sexual function and satisfaction:

Erectile Dysfunction: In men, increased sugar intake and the resulting insulin resistance and hyperglycemia might lead to erectile dysfunction (ED). ED is generally a result of reduced blood flow to the penis, which can be caused by vascular damage from prolonged high blood sugar levels. The endothelial cells that line the blood arteries can be harmed by high glucose levels, limiting the production of nitric oxide, a chemical that relaxes blood vessels and improves blood flow. Without sufficient nitric oxide, establishing and sustaining an erection becomes difficult.

Reduced Libido: Both men and women may notice a drop in libido (sexual desire) owing to increased sugar intake. Insulin resistance and metabolic syndrome are connected with hormonal abnormalities, including lower levels of testosterone, a critical hormone in sexual desire and function. Elevated insulin levels can also enhance the development of sex hormone-binding globulin (SHBG), a protein that binds to sex hormones and limits their availability, further lowering libido.

Vaginal Health: In women, increased sugar intake can contribute to vaginal health issues that influence sexual function and comfort. High blood sugar levels can raise the risk of yeast infections (candidiasis) and bacterial vaginosis, both of which can cause pain, itching, and discharge. These disorders can make sexual activity painful and diminish sexual enjoyment.

Hormonal Imbalances: High sugar intake can disturb the balance of important hormones involved in sexual health, including insulin, testosterone, estrogen, and cortisol. Insulin resistance can lead to higher cortisol levels (the stress hormone), which can severely impair sexual desire and performance. Additionally, hormonal imbalances can influence menstrual regularity and reproductive health in women, leading to disorders such as polycystic ovarian syndrome (PCOS), which is characterized by irregular periods, infertility, and symptoms such as hirsutism (excessive hair growth).

Mental Health and Stress: Excess sugar consumption is associated with poor mental health outcomes, including increased risk of depression and anxiety. Mental health is strongly tied to sexual health since psychological well-being has a key impact on sexual desire, arousal, and satisfaction. High sugar intake can increase stress and mental disorders, lowering overall quality of life and sexual health.

Energy Levels and Stamina: Chronic high sugar intake can lead to swings in blood sugar levels, resulting in periods of hyperglycemia followed by hypoglycemia (low blood sugar). These swings can produce weariness, weakness, and lower energy levels, all of which can severely impair sexual performance and satisfaction. Stable energy levels are vital for maintaining stamina and engaging in fulfilling sexual activity.

Chapter 2

The Physiology of Sexual Health

When it comes to human well-being, sexual health is a comprehensive component that encompasses not only the physical level but also the emotional and psychological levels. It is an extremely important factor in both general health and the quality of life. To gain an understanding of the physiology of sexual health, it is necessary to investigate how the many systems in the body collaborate to preserve sexual function and desire. Having a healthy sexual experience is dependent on several factors, including hormones, blood flow, nerve function, and mental wellness. This chapter explores the physiological foundations of sexual health, including how blood sugar levels can affect sexual function and libido, as well as the numerous components that make up sexual health.

Overview of Sexual Health

Sexual health is described by the World Health Organization (WHO) as a condition of physical, emotional, mental, and social well-being associated with sexuality. It is not simply the absence of disease, dysfunction, or infirmity; rather, it is an approach to sexuality and sexual interactions that is positive and respectful. Having a positive and respectful attitude about sexuality and sexual interactions is necessary for good sexual health. Additionally, it is essential to have the opportunity to have sexual encounters that are both joyful and safe, free from any form of coercion, discrimination, or violence.

Several factors contribute to sexual health:

Physical Health: The body's ability to function properly, including the reproductive system, cardiovascular health, hormonal balance, and overall physical fitness.

Emotional and Psychological Health: Emotional stability, mental health, and the ability to manage stress and anxiety play key roles in sexual health. Desire, performance, and satisfaction in sexual encounters are all influenced by psychological well-being.

Social and Relationship Factors: Healthy, respectful, and consensual relationships are crucial to sexual wellness. Communication, trust, and mutual respect between partners are vital.

Sexual Rights: The right to sexual health, including access to information, education, and services, as well as the right to consensual sexual activity and the freedom to express one's sexuality.

How Blood Sugar Levels Affect Libido and Sexual Function

Blood sugar levels can have a profound impact on sexual function and libido. Both hyperglycemia (high blood sugar) and hypoglycemia (low blood sugar) can disturb the normal physiological processes necessary for good sexual performance.

Hyperglycemia and Sexual Health

Hyperglycemia, commonly connected with diabetes, can lead to various issues that influence sexual health:

Blood Vessel Damage: Elevated blood sugar levels can damage blood vessels, affecting blood flow to numerous regions of the body, including the vaginal area. Adequate blood flow is needed for arousal and establishing and maintaining an erection in men and lubrication in women.

Nerve Damage (Neuropathy): Chronic high blood sugar can damage nerves, especially those involved in sexual arousal and response. Diabetic neuropathy can result in decreased feeling, reduced enjoyment, and erectile dysfunction in men.

Inflammation: Chronic inflammation produced by excessive blood sugar can damage several body systems, including those involved in sexual function.

Inflammation can cause pain and discomfort during intercourse, limiting sexual desire and satisfaction.

Hypoglycemia and Sexual Health

Hypoglycemia, or low blood sugar, can also negatively affect sexual health:

Energy Levels: Low blood sugar can lead to weariness and low energy levels, limiting the desire for sexual activity. Feeling physically fatigued can limit interest in sex and affect performance.

Mood and Mental Health: Hypoglycemia can produce mood swings, impatience, and anxiety, which can interfere with sexual desire and performance. Stable mental health is vital for a strong sexual relationship.

Physical Symptoms: Symptoms of hypoglycemia, including dizziness, perspiration, and confusion, can disturb intimate moments and make sexual activity uncomfortable or risky.

Maintaining steady blood sugar levels is vital for preserving sexual health and function. Effective management of blood sugar through food, exercise, and medication can help offset the detrimental effects of hyperglycemia and hypoglycemia on sexual health.

Components of Sexual Health

Sexual health is determined by a complex interplay of physical, emotional, and psychological factors. Each component is crucial to the entire experience of sexual health and well-being.

Physical Components

The physical components of sexual health include the proper functioning of the reproductive system, hormonal balance, cardiovascular health, and overall physical fitness.

Reproductive System: The health of the reproductive organs is vital for sexual function. For men, it includes the penis, testes, and prostate. For women, it involves the vagina, ovaries, uterus, and clitoris. Any dysfunction or disease affecting these organs can damage sexual health.

Hormonal Balance: Hormones such as testosterone, estrogen, and progesterone play key roles in sexual desire and function. Imbalances in these hormones can contribute to difficulties such as diminished libido, erectile dysfunction, and menstrual abnormalities.

Cardiovascular Health: Good cardiovascular health promotes enough blood flow to the vaginal area, which is crucial for arousal and sexual performance. Conditions such as hypertension and atherosclerosis can decrease blood flow and influence sexual health.

Physical health: General physical health contributes to stamina, energy levels, and overall well-being, all of which are necessary for a good sexual life. Regular exercise can enhance sexual performance and increase libido.

Emotional Components

Emotional health greatly influences sexual health. Emotional stability, the ability to manage stress, and high self-esteem are necessary for a healthy sexual experience.

Emotional Stability: Being emotionally stable and able to manage stress and anxiety favorably improves sexual desire and performance. Emotional turmoil can limit interest in sex and lead to concerns such as erectile dysfunction or difficulties in arousal.

Self-Esteem and Body Image: Positive self-esteem and a healthy body image led to confidence in sexual relationships. Feeling good about oneself and one's body promotes sexual desire and satisfaction.

Closeness and Connection: Emotional closeness and a deep connection with a partner generate a great sexual encounter. Trust, communication, and emotional support are vital to a healthy sexual relationship.

Psychological Components

Psychological health comprises mental well-being, cognitive function, and the ability to experience pleasure and satisfaction.

Mental Well-being: Good mental health is crucial for a good sexual life. Conditions such as depression, anxiety, and other mental health conditions can significantly impair sexual desire and function.

Cognitive Function: Cognitive talents, particularly attention and concentration, play a role in sexual desire and performance. Distractions or cognitive deficiencies can interfere with sexual satisfaction.

Pleasure and Satisfaction: The ability to experience pleasure and satisfaction is a fundamental component of sexual health. Psychological factors, including prior experiences, cultural beliefs, and personal attitudes toward sex, might influence one's ability to enjoy and get satisfaction from sexual engagement.

How Blood Sugar Levels Affect Hormone Balance and Neurotransmitter Function

Blood sugar levels, also known as blood glucose levels, play a key role in maintaining the body's overall homeostasis, particularly regulating hormone balance and neurotransmitter function. Glucose is the main energy source for the body and the brain, and its levels need to be strictly regulated. When blood sugar levels are continuously high (hyperglycemia) or low (hypoglycemia), it can lead to a disruption in hormone production and neurotransmitter activity, impacting several body functions, including sexual health.

The Role of Hormones and Neurotransmitters in Sexual Health

Hormones and neurotransmitters are vital for controlling several physiological functions, including sexual function and libido. Hormones are chemical messengers created by endocrine glands and are released into the bloodstream to target certain organs. Neurotransmitters, on the other hand, are chemical compounds that carry messages across synapses from one neuron to another in the nervous system. Both hormones and neurotransmitters interact to govern sexual arousal, desire, and performance.

Key Hormones in Sexual Health

Testosterone: Often connected with male sexual health, testosterone is equally significant in females. It is vital for libido, and erectile function in men, and arousal in women. Testosterone levels naturally fall with age, but imbalances can also emerge from health issues, particularly those caused by blood sugar levels.

Estrogen and Progesterone: These are the primary female sex hormones that regulate the menstrual cycle, reproductive system, and sexual desire. Estrogen is vital for maintaining vaginal lubrication and suppleness, whereas progesterone helps balance the effects of estrogen and is involved in mood control.

Oxytocin: Known as the "love hormone," oxytocin is released during physical touch, sexual activity, and childbirth. It enhances connection, emotional connection, and sexual satisfaction.

Prolactin: While prolactin is generally known for its involvement in lactation, it also promotes sexual enjoyment. High amounts of prolactin might diminish libido.

Cortisol: This stress hormone can have a substantial impact on sexual health. High cortisol levels, frequently stemming from persistent stress, might decrease sexual desire and performance.

Key Neurotransmitters in Sexual Health

Dopamine: This neurotransmitter is related to pleasure and reward. It has a role in sexual arousal and orgasm. Low dopamine levels might lead to lower sexual desire and fulfillment.

Serotonin: Serotonin helps regulate mood, and high amounts might suppress sexual desire. Antidepressant drugs that raise serotonin levels can sometimes contribute to sexual dysfunction.

Norepinephrine: This neurotransmitter is involved in the body's fight-or-flight response and can improve sexual arousal and desire.

Endorphins: These natural painkillers and mood enhancers are released during physical exertion and sexual activity, adding to sensations of pleasure and well-being.

The Impact of Blood Sugar on Hormones and Neurotransmitters

Maintaining steady blood sugar levels is critical for the efficient functioning of hormones and neurotransmitters. Fluctuations in blood glucose can lead to hormonal imbalances and changes in neurotransmitter activity, severely compromising sexual health.

Hyperglycemia and Hormonal Imbalance

Hyperglycemia can develop into insulin resistance, a disease when cells do not respond adequately to insulin. This can produce numerous hormonal imbalances, including:

Insulin and Testosterone: Insulin resistance can diminish testosterone levels in men, leading to reduced libido and erectile dysfunction. In women, insulin resistance is connected with polycystic ovarian syndrome (PCOS), which can cause irregular menstrual cycles, hirsutism, and infertility.

Estrogen and Progesterone: Hyperglycemia can disturb the balance of estrogen and progesterone in women, resulting in monthly abnormalities, diminished sexual desire, and issues with arousal and lubrication.

Cortisol: Chronic hyperglycemia can increase cortisol levels, leading to stress and its related detrimental consequences on sexual health, such as diminished libido and erectile dysfunction.

Hypoglycemia and Neurotransmitter Disruption

Hypoglycemia, or low blood sugar, can disrupt neurotransmitter activity, leading to mood swings, irritability, and anxiety, which can all severely affect sexual health.

Dopamine and Serotonin: Low blood sugar can lower dopamine levels, limiting sexual desire and pleasure. It can also induce variations in serotonin levels, leading to mood disorders and decreased libido.

Norepinephrine and Endorphins: Hypoglycemia can lead to a drop in norepinephrine and endorphin levels, resulting in diminished arousal and sensations of pleasure during sexual activity.

Hormonal Influences on Sexual Health

Hormones have a vital role in controlling sexual health and function. Imbalances in hormone levels can contribute to various sexual health disorders, underscoring the need to maintain hormonal balance for optimal sexual well-being.

Testosterone

Testosterone is necessary for both male and female sexual health. It influences libido, sexual desire, and performance. Low testosterone levels in men can contribute to erectile dysfunction, lower sexual desire, and poor sexual satisfaction. In women, low testosterone can result in diminished libido and difficulty with arousal and orgasm. Maintaining regulated testosterone levels is vital for a healthy sexual life.

Estrogen and Progesterone

In women, estrogen and progesterone regulate the menstrual cycle, reproductive system, and sexual desire. Estrogen is vital for maintaining vaginal health, including lubrication and suppleness. Low estrogen levels can contribute to vaginal dryness, pain during intercourse, and decreased libido. Progesterone helps balance the effects of estrogen and is important in mood control. Imbalances in these hormones can contribute to menstrual abnormalities, mood swings, and sexual

Prolactin

Prolactin is primarily known for its involvement in lactation, but it also promotes sexual enjoyment. High amounts of prolactin might impair libido and sexual desire. In some circumstances, excessive prolactin levels might lead to sexual dysfunction. Maintaining normal prolactin levels is vital for sexual health and happiness.

Cortisol

Cortisol, the body's major stress hormone, can have a substantial impact on sexual health. Chronic stress and increased cortisol levels can decrease sexual desire and performance. High cortisol levels can contribute to diminished libido, erectile dysfunction, and difficulty with arousal and orgasm. Managing stress and maintaining normal cortisol levels is vital for a healthy sexual life.

Key Hormones Involved in Sexual Function

Sexual function is controlled by a complicated interaction of hormones that determine desire, arousal, performance, and satisfaction. Understanding the roles of important hormones in sexual health can provide insights into how imbalances may impair sexual function and general well-being.

Erectile Function: In men, testosterone is necessary for erectile function. It boosts the synthesis of nitric oxide, a chemical that relaxes blood vessels and improves blood flow to the penis, enabling erections. Low testosterone levels might contribute to erectile dysfunction (ED).

Muscular Mass and Strength: Testosterone supports the development and maintenance of muscular mass and strength, which can improve general physical health and endurance, indirectly influencing sexual performance.

Mood and Energy Levels: Testosterone affects mood and energy levels, with low levels generally connected with weariness, depression, and irritability, all of which can severely impact sexual function.

Vaginal Health: Estrogen is vital for preserving the health of the vaginal tissues. It increases lubrication, flexibility, and thickness of the vaginal lining, minimizing discomfort during intercourse.

Menstrual Cycle and Reproductive Health: Estrogen governs the menstrual cycle and is vital for reproductive health. Imbalances can lead to irregular periods, impacting sexual health and fertility.

Bone Health: Estrogen helps maintain bone density, which is crucial for overall health and physical activity, indirectly influencing sexual health.

Progesterone

Progesterone is another crucial hormone in female sexual health, produced in the ovaries following ovulation and by the placenta during pregnancy.

Regulation of Menstrual Cycle: Progesterone helps regulate the menstrual cycle and prepare the body for prospective pregnancy. It balances the effects of estrogen and maintains reproductive health.

Mood and Well-being: Progesterone has relaxing effects and can influence mood. Imbalances may lead to mood swings and anxiety, which can influence sexual desire and fulfillment.

Pregnancy Support: Progesterone is vital for maintaining pregnancy, promoting the development of the uterine lining, and preventing premature labor.

Oxytocin

Oxytocin, frequently refers to as "love hormone," is produced in the hypothalamus and released by the pituitary gland.

Bonding and Emotional Connection: Oxytocin is released during physical touch, sexual activity, and childbirth, fostering bonding and emotional connection between partners.

Sexual Pleasure: Oxytocin improves feelings of sexual pleasure and contentment. It is released during orgasm, adding to the sense of intimacy and connection with a partner.

Sexual Satisfaction: Prolactin levels rise after orgasm and are thought to play a role in the refractory period, the time following orgasm during which it is difficult to achieve another orgasm.

Libido: High amounts of prolactin might diminish libido. Conditions that raise prolactin, such as some pituitary tumors, can lead to diminished sexual desire and satisfaction.

Stress Response: Chronic stress and increased cortisol levels might impair sexual desire and performance. High cortisol can contribute to diminished libido, erectile dysfunction, and issues with arousal and orgasm.

Energy and Mood: Cortisol regulates energy levels and mood. Imbalances can lead to exhaustion, anxiety, and sadness, all of which can significantly impact sexual health.

Physical Factors Affecting Sexual Health

Sexual health is regulated by a multitude of physical elements, including blood flow, nerve function, and overall physiological health. These components are crucial for the regular functioning of the reproductive system and the sense of sexual pleasure and fulfillment.

Blood Flow

Adequate blood flow is vital for sexual pleasure and performance. Blood flow is required for establishing and sustaining erections in men and for lubrication and sensitivity in women.

Erectile Function in Men: Erections develop when blood flows into the penile tissues, causing them to enlarge and become stiff. Conditions that decrease blood flow, such as atherosclerosis, hypertension, and diabetes, can contribute to erectile dysfunction.

Lubrication and Sensitivity in Women: Blood flow to the vaginal tissues is necessary for lubrication and sensitivity. Reduced blood flow can lead to vaginal dryness and pain during intercourse.

Cardiovascular Health: Overall cardiovascular health plays a key role in ensuring proper blood flow. Regular exercise, a good diet, and treating illnesses like hypertension and high cholesterol are vital for sexual health.

Nerve Function

Nerve function is necessary for the transfer of impulses between the brain and the reproductive organs, permitting arousal, sensation, and orgasm.

Neuropathy: Conditions such as diabetes can lead to neuropathy, or nerve damage, which can affect sexual function. Diabetic neuropathy can produce decreased feeling and impaired sexual satisfaction.

Spinal Cord Injuries: Injuries to the spinal cord can alter the neurological pathways involved in sexual function, leading to difficulties with arousal and orgasm.

Mental Health: Psychological variables, including stress, anxiety, and depression, can alter nerve function and the brain's ability to process sexual cues, resulting in lower sexual desire and performance.

Hormonal Balance

Hormonal balance is vital for maintaining sexual wellness. Imbalances in hormones such as testosterone, estrogen, and progesterone can contribute to numerous sexual health disorders.

Hormonal Imbalances in Men: Low testosterone levels can contribute to lower libido, erectile dysfunction, and decreased sexual satisfaction. Conditions such as hypogonadism, when the testes produce inadequate testosterone, can influence sexual health.

Hormonal Imbalances in Women: Imbalances in estrogen and progesterone can contribute to monthly abnormalities, lower libido, and difficulty with arousal and lubrication. Conditions such as PCOS and menopause can dramatically impair hormonal balance and sexual health.

Physical Fitness

Overall physical fitness contributes to stamina, energy levels, and general well-being, all of which are crucial for a good sexual life.

Exercise: Regular physical activity improves cardiovascular health, enhances blood flow, and helps maintain a healthy weight, all of which support sexual performance. Exercise also releases endorphins, which increase mood and reduce stress.

Weight Management: Maintaining a healthy weight is important for sexual health. Obesity is related to a higher risk of illnesses such as diabetes, hypertension, and cardiovascular disease, which can affect sexual performance.

Nutrition: A balanced diet rich in nutrients improves general health and hormonal equilibrium. Specific minerals, such as zinc and omega-3 fatty acids, play roles in supporting sexual health.

Sleep:

Adequate sleep is vital for maintaining energy levels, hormone balance, and overall health, all of which contribute to sexual function and satisfaction.

Hormonal Regulation: Sleep is vital for the regulation of hormones such as testosterone and cortisol. Disrupted sleep habits can lead to hormone imbalances, compromising sexual health.

Energy and Mood: Quality sleep boosts mental and physical energy levels, lowering weariness and increasing mood. Poor sleep can lead to irritation, anxiety, and sadness, negatively affecting sexual desire and performance.

Blood Flow, Nerve Function, and Other Physiological Aspects

The physiological components of sexual health extend beyond hormones and involve numerous systems working together to support sexual function and happiness.

Blood Flow

Adequate blood flow to the vaginal area is vital for sexual pleasure and performance. In men, erections are based on the ability of blood to flow into and fill the penile tissues. In women, blood flow to the vaginal and clitoral tissues is crucial for lubrication and sensitivity.

Nitric Oxide and Blood Flow: Nitric oxide is a chemical that plays a vital role in vasodilation, and the widening of blood vessels. It is secreted during sexual stimulation and increases blood flow to the vaginal area, increasing erections in men and boosting sensitivity and lubrication in women.

Vascular Health: Conditions that compromise vascular health, such as atherosclerosis and hypertension, can limit blood flow and lead to sexual dysfunction. Maintaining healthy blood vessels through nutrition, exercise, and treating illnesses like hypertension and diabetes is vital for sexual health.

Nerve Function

Nerve function is crucial for delivering messages between the brain and the reproductive organs, permitting arousal, sensation, and orgasm.

Peripheral Nerves: Peripheral nerves carry sensory information from the genital area to the brain and movement impulses from the brain to the genital area. Damage to these nerves, such as from diabetes or spinal cord injury, can impede sexual function.

Central Nervous System: The central nervous system, including the brain and spinal cord, processes sexual cues and coordinates the bodily reactions of arousal and orgasm. Mental health problems, such as anxiety and depression, can influence the brain's ability to process sexual impulses, resulting in diminished sexual desire and performance.

Muscular Function

Muscular function, particularly in the pelvic floor, plays a key influence on sexual health.

Pelvic Floor Muscles: Strong pelvic floor muscles support the pelvic organs, promote sexual pleasure, and contribute to the ability to produce and maintain erections in men and vaginal tightness in women. Pelvic floor exercises, such as Kegels, can strengthen these muscles and improve sexual function.

Muscle Tone and Flexibility: Overall muscle tone and flexibility contribute to stamina and physical comfort during sexual activity. Regular exercise and stretching can improve muscle function and boost sexual performance.

Endocrine Function

The endocrine system, which creates and regulates hormones, is crucial to sexual health. Hormonal imbalances can lead to several sexual health disorders.

Thyroid Function: Thyroid hormones influence metabolism and energy levels. Hypothyroidism (underactive thyroid) and hyperthyroidism (overactive thyroid) can contribute to changes in libido, erectile dysfunction, and menstrual abnormalities.

Adrenal Function: The adrenal glands generate cortisol, adrenaline, and other chemicals that regulate stress response and energy levels. Chronic stress and adrenal exhaustion can lead to diminished sexual desire and performance.

Overall Health

Overall health and well-being are vital to sexual health. Conditions that impair general health might also impact sexual function.

Chronic Illnesses: Chronic illnesses such as diabetes, cardiovascular disease, and autoimmune disorders might impact sexual health. Managing these problems through medical therapy and lifestyle adjustments is critical for sustaining sexual function.

Mental Health: Mental health is intimately linked to sexual health. Conditions such as anxiety, sadness, and stress can impair sexual desire and performance. Seeking treatment for mental health disorders can improve sexual well-being.

Lifestyle Factors: Lifestyle factors, including food, exercise, sleep, and stress management, play essential roles in sustaining general health and sexual performance. Healthy lifestyle choices encourage hormonal balance, vascular health, and mental well-being, all of which lead to a pleasant sexual life.

Understanding the functions of hormones, physical variables, and physiological features in sexual health is vital for maintaining a healthy and gratifying sexual life. By treating imbalances and managing underlying health issues, individuals can boost their sexual performance and general well-being.

Chapter 3

How Blood Sugar Levels Affect Sexual Health

Blood sugar levels have a substantial impact on sexual health, influencing a range of physiological processes and general well-being. Both high and low blood sugar levels can affect sexual function, desire, and satisfaction, making glucose regulation a key element of sustaining sexual health. This section dives into the mechanisms by which blood sugar levels affect sexual health and the broader implications for reproductive health and general quality of life.

How High Blood Sugar Affects Sexual Health
Erectile Dysfunction in Men

High blood sugar levels are closely connected with erectile dysfunction (ED) in men. Persistent hyperglycemia can damage blood vessels and nerves, leading to impaired blood flow and nerve function, both of which are necessary for establishing and sustaining an erection. The endothelial cells that line the blood vessels can be particularly sensitive to injury from high glucose levels, limiting the production of nitric oxide. Nitric oxide is a key chemical that helps blood vessels relax, allowing increased blood flow necessary for an erection.

Without sufficient nitric oxide, the ability to achieve and maintain an erection is greatly reduced.

Reduced Libido

Hyperglycemia can lead to hormonal imbalances that impact libido in both men and women. High insulin levels can decrease the production of sex hormones such as testosterone, which plays a vital role in sexual desire. Additionally, high blood sugar can increase levels of sex hormone-binding globulin (SHBG), which binds to sex hormones and makes them less available to the body's tissues. This decline in bioavailable testosterone might lower libido, resulting in diminished sexual desire and satisfaction.

Vaginal Health in Women

For women, elevated blood sugar levels might contribute to vaginal health concerns that influence sexual function and comfort. Elevated glucose levels generate an environment susceptible to yeast infections (candidiasis) and bacterial vaginosis. These disorders can cause itching, discomfort, and discharge, making sexual activity uncomfortable and limiting sexual satisfaction. Chronic high blood sugar can also lead to a disease known as diabetic neuropathy, which can cause nerve damage and impair sensitivity in the vaginal area, further reducing sexual pleasure.

Orgasmic Function

Both men and women may encounter difficulty with orgasm as a result of elevated blood sugar levels. Neuropathy, a common symptom of diabetes, can impair feeling in the vaginal area, making it harder to attain orgasm. Additionally, vascular damage from continuous hyperglycemia can limit blood flow to the genitals, lowering the physical responses necessary for orgasm. This can lead to frustration, diminished sexual satisfaction, and pressure on intimate relationships.

How High Blood Sugar Affects Fertility in Both Men and Women

High blood sugar levels can have major effects on fertility, influencing both men and women through numerous processes.

Male Fertility

High blood sugar levels can severely impair male fertility in numerous ways. Elevated glucose levels can impede spermatogenesis, the process by which sperm are generated. This can lead to lower sperm count, poor sperm motility, and aberrant sperm morphology. These conditions can decrease the likelihood of successful fertilization.

Additionally, oxidative stress, which is heightened by hyperglycemia, can damage sperm DNA, lowering sperm quality and raising the chance of miscarriage and genetic defects in kids. Insulin resistance and metabolic syndrome, commonly associated with high blood sugar levels, can also contribute to reduced testosterone levels, further compromising fertility by lowering desire and sexual performance.

Female Fertility

In women, elevated blood sugar levels can disrupt menstrual cycles and ovulation, making it more difficult to conceive. Hyperglycemia can lead to hormonal imbalances that alter the regularity of menstrual periods. For example, insulin resistance can increase the amounts of insulin and androgens (male hormones) in the body, leading to illnesses such as polycystic ovarian syndrome (PCOS). PCOS is characterized by irregular menstrual periods, anovulation (lack of ovulation), and symptoms such as hirsutism (excessive hair growth). These hormonal changes might make it difficult for women to forecast their reproductive periods and achieve conception.

High blood sugar levels can also alter the endometrial lining of the uterus, making it less susceptible to embryo implantation. This can lead to reduced implantation rates and a higher risk of early pregnancy loss. Furthermore, increased glucose levels can generate an inflammatory milieu in the reproductive tract, further affecting fertility.

Role of Inflammation and Advanced Glycation End Products (AGEs)

Inflammation and advanced glycation end products (AGEs) are major variables in the adverse impact of high blood sugar levels on sexual health and fertility.

Inflammation

Chronic inflammation is a characteristic of hyperglycemia and insulin resistance. High blood sugar levels induce pro-inflammatory cytokines and other inflammatory mediators, which can harm tissues and organs, including those involved in sexual and reproductive health. Inflammation can compromise endothelial function, lowering blood flow to the genitals and contributing to erectile dysfunction in men and diminished arousal in women.

Inflammation can also affect the precise hormonal balance essential for good reproductive function. For example, inflammatory cytokines can interfere with the hypothalamic-pituitary-gonadal (HPG) axis, which governs the production of sex hormones such as testosterone, estrogen, and progesterone. This disruption can lead to hormonal abnormalities that impact libido, sexual function, and fertility.

Advanced Glycation End Products (AGEs)

AGEs are toxic chemicals that arise when proteins or lipids intermingle with sugar in the bloodstream through glycation. High blood sugar levels stimulate the development of AGEs, which can accumulate in many tissues and organs, causing damage and dysfunction.

AGEs can cross-link with collagen and elastin fibers in blood vessels, diminishing their elasticity and limiting blood flow. This arterial damage is a crucial element in the development of erectile dysfunction and other vascular-related sexual health concerns. AGEs can also destroy nerve cells, resulting in neuropathy and diminished feeling in the vaginal area.

In the reproductive system, AGEs can impact ovarian and testicular function, limiting fertility. In women, AGEs can disturb the ovarian environment, compromising the quality of oocytes (eggs) and the function of granulosa cells, which are required for follicle formation and hormone synthesis. In men, AGEs can harm the seminiferous tubules, where sperm are generated, leading to diminished sperm quality and quantity.

Moreover, AGEs can promote oxidative stress and inflammation, further worsening their adverse effects on sexual health and fertility. Oxidative stress arises when there is an imbalance between the creation of reactive oxygen species (free radicals) and the body's antioxidant defenses. This imbalance can damage cellular components, including DNA, proteins, and lipids, leading to cellular malfunction and death.

Specific Impacts on Reproductive Organs: Ovaries, Endometrium, and Sperm

The effects of elevated blood sugar levels extend to several reproductive organs, including the ovaries, endometrium, and sperm. These consequences can profoundly change reproductive health, fertility, and overall sexual function.

Ovaries

The ovaries are vital for female reproductive health, generating oocytes (eggs) and releasing sex hormones such as estrogen and progesterone. Elevated blood sugar levels can interfere with ovarian function in several ways:

Hormonal Imbalances: High blood sugar can lead to insulin resistance, which can increase the production of insulin and androgens (male hormones) in women. These hormonal abnormalities are symptomatic of disorders like polycystic ovarian syndrome (PCOS). PCOS affects a high number of women of reproductive age and is associated with irregular menstrual periods, anovulation (lack of ovulation), and infertility. The excess insulin and androgens impair normal ovarian function, resulting in the development of numerous cysts in the ovaries.

Oocyte Quality: High blood sugar levels might negatively impair the quality of oocytes. Hyperglycemia can generate a hazardous environment for developing oocytes, leading to oxidative stress and damage. Poor oocyte quality can diminish the chances of successful fertilization and raise the risk of genetic disorders in the embryo.

Follicular Development: The follicular environment, where oocytes mature, is similarly influenced by elevated blood sugar levels. Elevated hyperglycemia can disrupt the activity of granulosa cells, which are crucial for the nutrition and maturation of the oocyte. This disruption can affect follicular development and ovulation, further lowering fertility.

Endometrium

The endometrium is the lining of the uterus that thickens in preparation for embryo implantation. High blood sugar levels can damage the endometrium in numerous ways:

Endometrial Receptivity: Hyperglycemia can alter the endometrial lining, making it less receptive to embryo implantation. Insulin resistance and inflammation linked to high blood sugar can affect the expression of essential molecules involved in implantation, lowering the likelihood of a successful pregnancy.

Menstrual Irregularities: Hormonal imbalances induced by high blood sugar levels might contribute to irregular menstrual periods. Irregular cycles might make it harder to predict ovulation and diminish the likelihood of a timely pregnancy. Additionally, monthly irregularities are commonly accompanied by disorders like PCOS, which further impede fertility.

Sperm

Male reproductive health is also strongly impacted by high blood sugar levels, specifically lowering sperm quality and function:

Sperm Count and Motility: Hyperglycemia can impede spermatogenesis, the process by which sperm are generated. This impairment can lead to a lower sperm count and poor sperm motility (the ability of sperm to move efficiently). Both factors are important for effective fertilization, and their reduction can lower fertility.

Sperm Morphology: High blood sugar levels can lead to aberrant sperm morphology, changing the form and structure of sperm. Abnormal sperm are less capable of fertilizing an egg, limiting the chances of conception.

DNA Damage: Elevated blood sugar levels can produce oxidative stress, resulting in DNA damage in sperm. Oxidative stress occurs from an imbalance between reactive oxygen species (ROS) and the body's antioxidant defenses. DNA damage in sperm can raise

the likelihood of genetic defects in the embryo and lead
to early pregnancy loss.

Impact on Men's Sexual Health

High blood sugar levels can have substantial
implications on men's sexual health, impacting different
areas of sexual function and general well-being.

Erectile Dysfunction (ED)

Erectile dysfunction is one of the most prevalent sexual
health disorders among men with high blood sugar
levels. ED occurs when a man is unable to start or
maintain an erection sufficient for satisfactory sexual
performance. Several variables contribute to ED in the
context of elevated blood sugar:

Vascular Damage: Chronic hyperglycemia can harm
blood vessels, decreasing blood flow to the penis. The
endothelial cells lining the blood vessels can be harmed
by high glucose levels, limiting the production of nitric
oxide. Nitric oxide is vital for relaxing blood vessels and
permitting greater blood flow necessary for an erection.
Without sufficient nitric oxide, attaining and sustaining
an erection becomes difficult.

Nerve Damage: High blood sugar levels can lead to
diabetic neuropathy, a disorder characterized by nerve
damage. Nerves that govern erection can be injured,
limiting sensitivity and the capacity to generate an

erection. Neuropathy can also produce pain and discomfort, further impairing sexual activity.

Libido and Sexual Desire

High blood sugar levels might impair libido and sexual desire in men:

Testosterone Levels: Testosterone is an important hormone in regulating sexual desire and function. High blood sugar levels can inhibit testosterone production and raise SHBG levels, leading to a decrease in bioavailable testosterone. This decline can impair libido and sexual desire.

Sperm Quality and Its Vulnerability to Inflammation

Sperm quality is critical for male fertility and is particularly vulnerable to the effects of inflammation and oxidative stress induced by high blood sugar levels.

Oxidative Stress: High blood sugar levels stimulate the generation of reactive oxygen species (ROS), resulting in oxidative stress. Oxidative stress can damage the DNA, proteins, and lipids in sperm, lowering their quality and function. Damaged sperm are less capable of fertilizing an egg and may raise the chance of genetic defects in progeny.

Inflammation: Hyperglycemia can produce inflammation in the reproductive system, altering the environment in which sperm form and function. Inflammatory cytokines can affect the normal function of Sertoli cells, which maintain and nourish growing sperm. This disturbance can impair spermatogenesis and diminish sperm quality.

DNA Integrity: Sperm DNA integrity is critical for successful fertilization and good embryonic development. High blood sugar levels can cause DNA fragmentation in sperm, leading to lower fertility and increased risk of miscarriage and genetic disorders. Maintaining normal blood sugar levels is critical for protecting sperm DNA integrity and overall reproductive health.

Seminal Fluid: The quality of seminal fluid, which nourishes and protects sperm, can also be altered by high blood sugar levels. Hyperglycemia can affect the composition of seminal fluid, lowering its protective characteristics and rendering sperm more sensitive to environmental stresses.

Addressing Male Sexual Health in the Context of Blood Sugar Control

Managing blood sugar levels is vital for preserving male sexual health and general well-being. Several techniques can help address the impact of elevated blood sugar on sexual function and fertility:

Diet and Nutrition: Adopting a balanced diet rich in whole foods, fruits, vegetables, lean meats, and healthy fats will help regulate blood sugar levels. Reducing the intake of sugary meals and beverages is vital for controlling hyperglycemia and its related consequences. Incorporating meals with a low glycemic index (GI) will assist in maintaining stable blood sugar levels and improve overall health.

Physical Activity: Regular physical activity is vital for regulating blood sugar levels and boosting cardiovascular health. Exercise can enhance insulin sensitivity, allowing the body to use glucose more effectively. Physical activity also increases healthy blood flow and minimizes the risk of vascular injury, which is vital for preserving erectile function and overall sexual health.

Weight Management: Maintaining a healthy weight is vital for managing blood sugar levels and minimizing the risk of insulin resistance. Excess weight, particularly around the belly, might contribute to hormonal imbalances and raise the risk of erectile dysfunction. Achieving and maintaining a healthy weight through diet and exercise can improve overall health and sexual performance.

Medical care: For people with diabetes or prediabetes, competent medical care is critical for regulating blood sugar levels. Medications such as metformin can help enhance insulin sensitivity and manage blood sugar levels. Regular monitoring of blood sugar levels and working closely with healthcare specialists can help prevent issues and preserve good health.

Mental Health Support: Addressing mental health is a crucial element of regulating blood sugar levels and preserving sexual health. Chronic stress, despair, and anxiety can aggravate hyperglycemia and significantly disrupt sexual function. Seeking support from mental health specialists and adopting stress-reducing strategies such as mindfulness, meditation, and therapy can enhance general well-being and sexual health.

Lifestyle adjustments: Making lifestyle adjustments such as quitting smoking, lowering alcohol use, and getting appropriate sleep can also help manage blood sugar levels and improve sexual health. Smoking and excessive alcohol intake can contribute to vascular damage and erectile dysfunction, while poor sleep can influence insulin sensitivity and overall health.

Erectile Dysfunction and Its Relation to Blood Sugar Levels

Erectile dysfunction (ED) is a widespread issue among men, particularly those with diabetes or high blood sugar levels. ED is described as the inability to attain or sustain an erection sufficient for satisfactory sexual performance. The link between blood sugar levels and erectile function is complex and involves several physiological systems.

Vascular Health and Blood Flow

One of the key variables relating high blood sugar levels to erectile dysfunction is vascular health. An erection depends on proper blood flow to the penile tissues, which is helped by the dilatation of blood vessels. Chronic hyperglycemia can harm the endothelial cells lining the blood vessels, decreasing their ability to produce nitric oxide, a chemical needed for vasodilation. Without sufficient nitric oxide, the blood vessels cannot relax effectively, reducing blood flow to the penis and making it difficult to establish or maintain an erection.

Psychological Factors

Psychological issues such as stress, worry, and depression are typically linked to both high blood sugar levels and erectile dysfunction. The stress of managing a chronic condition like diabetes can contribute to mental health concerns, which in turn can influence sexual desire and performance. The anxiety surrounding sexual performance can create a cycle of concern and failure, aggravating erectile dysfunction.

Other Sexual Health Issues in Men

While erectile dysfunction is a big worry, excessive blood sugar levels can also damage other elements of male sexual health, including libido and ejaculation problems.

Hormonal Imbalances: As discussed previously, excessive blood sugar levels can lead to elevated insulin and SHBG, lowering bioavailable testosterone. Testosterone is a vital hormone in regulating libido, and lower levels can diminish sexual desire.

Ejaculation Problems

High blood sugar levels can also induce different ejaculation difficulties, including:

Delayed Ejaculation: Men with high blood sugar levels may experience delayed ejaculation, when there is a protracted period before ejaculation occurs. This issue can be frustrating and impact sexual satisfaction for both couples.

Retrograde Ejaculation: Retrograde ejaculation happens when semen enters the bladder instead of escaping from the penis during ejaculation. This illness is commonly connected with nerve damage caused by excessive blood sugar levels. Although not hazardous, retrograde ejaculation can lead to infertility and poor sexual satisfaction.

Premature Ejaculation: High blood sugar levels can also contribute to premature ejaculation, where ejaculation occurs sooner than anticipated during sexual activity. This syndrome can be connected to anxiety, stress, and other psychological aspects associated with controlling chronic hyperglycemia.

Sperm Motility

Sperm motility refers to the capacity of sperm to move efficiently through the female reproductive tract to reach and fertilize an egg. High blood sugar levels can affect sperm motility through numerous pathways, including:

Oxidative Damage: As with sperm count, oxidative stress can damage the structures of sperm, especially the mitochondria, which are critical for delivering the energy required for movement. Damaged mitochondria can limit the energy available to sperm, hindering their motility.

Inflammatory Environment: Inflammation in the reproductive tract can produce a hostile environment for sperm, decreasing their motility. Inflammatory cytokines can affect the composition of seminal fluid, diminishing its protective characteristics and making it more difficult for sperm to migrate properly.

Structural Abnormalities: High blood sugar levels can induce structural abnormalities in sperm, limiting their ability to swim properly. Abnormal sperm morphology can result from oxidative stress and hormonal abnormalities, lowering their motility and the likelihood of successful fertilization.

Sperm Morphology

Sperm morphology refers to the size and form of semen. Normal sperm have a streamlined shape with an oval head and a long tail, helping them to swim efficiently. High blood sugar levels can induce changes in sperm morphology, compromising fertility:

Protein Glycation: Advanced glycation end products (AGEs), which come from high blood sugar levels, can change proteins in sperm, changing their structure and function. Protein glycation can lead to aberrant sperm morphology, limiting their capacity to fertilize an egg.

Hormonal Effects: Hormonal imbalances caused by high blood sugar levels might alter the growth of sperm, resulting in abnormalities in size and form. Elevated insulin and changed testosterone levels can impair the maturation process of sperm, resulting in morphological abnormalities.

Impact on Women's Sexual Health

It is important to note that the influence of blood sugar levels on the sexual health of women is diverse and considerable. Several elements of reproductive health can be disrupted by elevated glucose levels, which can lead to problems that influence sexual function as well as overall well-being. A solid understanding of these effects is necessary to effectively address and manage the difficulties that women with high blood sugar levels may have.

Ovarian Function and

Irregular Ovulation

When blood sugar levels are high, ovarian function is one of the primary regions negatively impacted. Eggs, also known as oocytes, are produced by the ovaries, which are also responsible for the secretion of hormones like estrogen and progesterone, which are essential for regulating the menstrual cycle and providing support for pregnancy. The following are some examples of how elevated glucose levels can interfere with these processes:

Insulin resistance, which is a common consequence of high blood sugar levels, is intimately associated with the development of polycystic ovary syndrome (PCOS). Insulin resistance is a common consequence of blood sugar levels that are high. Multiple cysts on the ovaries, irregular menstrual cycles, and increased levels of androgens (male hormones) are features that are characteristic of polycystic ovary syndrome (PCOS). Insulin resistance can make these symptoms worse by elevating insulin and testosterone levels, which in turn disrupts the equilibrium of reproductive hormones. This hormonal imbalance can lead to irregular ovulation or anovulation (lack of ovulation), making it difficult for women to conceive.

Hormonal Imbalances: High blood sugar levels might alter the delicate balance of reproductive hormones. Insulin resistance can lead to greater insulin levels, which can enhance androgen production. Elevated androgens can block the release of follicle-stimulating hormone (FSH) and luteinizing hormone (LH), which are necessary for the maturation and release of eggs. This disruption might result in irregular or absent ovulation, lowering fertility.

Oxidative Stress: Hyperglycemia can lead to increased generation of reactive oxygen species (ROS), causing oxidative stress. Oxidative stress can harm the ovarian follicles where eggs develop, reducing their maturation and quality. This damage can result in fewer viable eggs being produced after ovulation, further lowering fertility.

Endometrial Health and Its Impact on Embryo Implantation

The endometrium, the inner lining of the uterus, plays a serious role in the menstrual cycle and pregnancy. It thickens in response to hormonal signals to prepare for the implantation of a fertilized egg. High blood sugar levels can severely affect endometrial health, influencing embryo implantation and pregnancy outcomes.

Endometrial Receptivity: For successful implantation, the endometrium must be receptive to the fertilized egg. Hyperglycemia can impair the hormonal signals that govern endometrial receptivity. Elevated insulin levels can lead to aberrant growth and development of the endometrial tissue, making it less suitable for implantation.

Inflammation: Chronic high blood sugar levels might produce inflammation in the endometrial tissue. Inflammatory cytokines can affect the expression of genes involved in endometrial receptivity, making it more difficult for the embryo to implant and establish a pregnancy. Inflammation can also lead to disorders such as endometriosis, when endometrial tissue grows outside the uterus, causing pain and infertility.

Glycation and Advanced Glycation End Products (AGEs): High blood sugar levels can lead to the production of AGEs, which are toxic chemicals that result from the non-enzymatic glycation of proteins and lipids. AGEs can accumulate in the endometrial tissue, altering its structure and function. These changes can compromise the endometrium's capacity to support implantation and early pregnancy, increasing the chance of miscarriage.

Vaginal Health and the Risk of Discomfort Due to Elevated Glucose Levels

Vaginal health is a vital element of women's sexual health, and increased glucose levels can significantly damage this area. The vagina has a delicate ecology that includes helpful bacteria, which help maintain a healthy pH and protect against infections. High blood sugar levels can upset this balance, leading to various complications.

Yeast Infections: Elevated glucose levels can produce an environment suitable for the growth of Candida, a kind of yeast that can cause infections. Yeast infections are characterized by itching, burning, and discharge, and they can greatly disrupt a woman's comfort and sexual activity. Women with high blood sugar levels are at an increased risk of recurring yeast infections, which can be tough to control and can damage sexual health and well-being.

Bacterial Vaginosis (BV): High blood sugar levels can also disturb the equilibrium of bacteria in the vagina, leading to bacterial vaginosis. BV develops when the balance of helpful and dangerous bacteria is interrupted, leading to symptoms such as discharge, odor, and irritation. BV can raise the risk of various infections and consequences, including pelvic inflammatory disease (PID) and bad pregnancy outcomes.

Dryness and Irritation: Hyperglycemia can contribute to vaginal dryness and irritation, which can cause pain during sexual activity. Vaginal dryness can arise from hormonal imbalances and inadequate lubrication, making intercourse unpleasant and lowering sexual satisfaction. Persistent dryness and irritation can lead to microtears and an increased risk of infection.

Blood sugar levels play a key role in regulating different body activities, including the menstrual cycle. The menstrual cycle is a complicated process driven by hormonal interactions, and any interruption in these hormones might lead to monthly abnormalities. Elevated blood sugar levels, particularly those linked with insulin resistance and diabetes, can dramatically influence menstrual health.

Hormonal Regulation of the Menstrual Cycle

The menstrual cycle is maintained by a precise balance of hormones, including estrogen, progesterone, follicle-stimulating hormone (FSH), and luteinizing hormone (LH). These hormones orchestrate the growing and release of an egg from the ovary, as well as the preparation of the endometrium for prospective implantation. Insulin, a hormone responsible for controlling blood sugar levels, also plays a critical part in this hormonal balance.

Insulin Resistance and Hormonal Imbalance: Insulin resistance, a disease where the body's cells do not respond adequately to insulin, can lead to high levels of insulin in the bloodstream. High insulin levels can alter the normal balance of reproductive hormones, leading to a rise in androgen levels. Elevated androgens can interfere with the regular release of FSH and LH, hormones required for the maturation and release of eggs from the ovaries. This disruption can result in irregular menstrual periods, anovulation (lack of ovulation), and disorders including polycystic ovarian syndrome (PCOS).

Hyperglycemia and Menstrual Irregularities: Persistently high blood sugar levels (hyperglycemia) might damage the hypothalamus and pituitary gland, which are crucial for regulating the menstrual cycle. Hyperglycemia can modify the secretion of gonadotropin-releasing hormone (GnRH) from the hypothalamus, which in turn alters the release of FSH and LH from the pituitary gland. This hormonal imbalance can lead to irregular or skipped periods, longer menstrual cycles, and severe bleeding.

Impact on Ovulation: High blood sugar levels can hinder ovulation by impairing the ovarian follicles' capacity to mature normally. This can result in fewer viable eggs being produced during ovulation, lowering fertility. Women with diabetes or insulin resistance may experience inconsistent ovulation, making it tough to anticipate their reproductive window and conceive.

Effects on the Luteal Phase: The luteal phase, the second half of the menstrual cycle following ovulation, is characterized by the production of progesterone, which prepares the endometrium for implantation. High blood sugar levels can damage the corpus luteum, the tissue that makes progesterone, leading to insufficient progesterone levels. This can result in luteal phase abnormalities, where the endometrium is not fully prepared for implantation, increasing the chance of early pregnancy loss.

Psychological and Emotional Effects

Blood sugar changes can have severe psychological and emotional repercussions, which in turn can impair sexual desire and general sexual health. The brain is particularly sensitive to fluctuations in glucose levels, and imbalances can contribute to mood swings, anxiety, sadness, and other emotional disorders.

Impact on Mood

Hypoglycemia and Mood Swings: Low blood sugar levels (hypoglycemia) can produce fast mood swings, anger, anxiety, and feelings of anxiousness. The brain relies on a regular supply of glucose to function efficiently, and when glucose levels decrease, it can stimulate the production of stress chemicals like adrenaline and cortisol. These hormones can lead to symptoms such as shakiness, perspiration, and an elevated heart rate, which can add to feelings of worry and panic.

Hyperglycemia and Depression: Chronic high blood sugar levels are related to an increased risk of depression. Hyperglycemia can lead to chronic inflammation and oxidative stress, which can disrupt brain function and contribute to the development of depressive symptoms. Additionally, the emotional strain of managing a chronic condition like diabetes can contribute to feelings of frustration, helplessness, and isolation, further worsening depression.

Blood Sugar Fluctuations and Emotional Stability: Fluctuations in blood sugar levels, whether related to hypoglycemia or hyperglycemia, can impair emotional stability. These changes might contribute to irritation, mood swings, and difficulties concentrating. For individuals with diabetes, maintaining stable blood sugar levels is critical for emotional well-being and mental health.

Impact on Sexual Desire

Hormonal Influence: Blood sugar levels can influence the generation and regulation of hormones that are crucial for sexual desire, such as testosterone and estrogen. Insulin resistance and high insulin levels can alter the usual balance of these hormones, resulting in a decrease in libido. For women, this can result in lower sexual desire and arousal, while men may notice a drop in libido and erectile function.

Energy Levels and Exhaustion: High blood sugar levels can contribute to chronic exhaustion, which can severely affect sexual desire and activity. Hyperglycemia can cause glucose to be expelled in the urine rather than being used by the body's cells for energy, resulting in sensations of fatigue and lethargy. Fatigue can limit the desire for sexual activities and make it challenging to engage in personal relationships.

Psychological Stress and Sexual Desire: The psychological stress involved with regulating blood sugar levels and dealing with the symptoms of diabetes might impair sexual desire. Stress can lead to the release of cortisol, a hormone that can reduce sexual desire. Additionally, the emotional toll of living with a chronic disease can lead to lower self-esteem and body image difficulties, further limiting sexual desire.

Impact on Relationship Dynamics: Blood sugar fluctuations can affect relationship dynamics, which can, in turn, impact sexual desire. Mood swings, impatience, and emotional instability can strain relationships, leading to disagreements and less closeness. Effective communication and support from partners are vital for handling the emotional issues associated with blood sugar variations and maintaining a successful sexual relationship.

Impact on Menstrual Health and Fertility

The association between blood sugar levels and menstrual cycles extends to fertility and reproductive health. Elevated blood sugar levels can contribute to irregular ovulation, making it difficult for women to conceive. Insulin resistance and hyperglycemia can also impact the quality of eggs and the condition of the endometrium, which are crucial for successful implantation and conception.

Ovulation and Egg Quality: High blood sugar levels might impede the maturation and release of eggs from the ovaries. This can result in fewer viable eggs being available for fertilization, lowering fertility. Additionally, oxidative stress caused by hyperglycemia can damage the ovarian follicles and decrease the quality of eggs, further reducing fertility.

Endometrial Health: The endometrium must be receptive to the fertilized egg for successful implantation. High blood sugar levels can affect the hormonal signals that regulate endometrial receptivity and promote inflammation, making it more difficult for the embryo to implant and establish a pregnancy. This can raise the risk of early pregnancy loss and problems.

Pregnancy Outcomes: Women with uncontrolled blood sugar levels are at a higher risk of difficulties during pregnancy, such as gestational diabetes, preeclampsia, and preterm birth. Proper management of blood sugar levels before and during pregnancy is vital for lowering these risks and ensuring a safe pregnancy.

Managing Stress and Anxiety Related to Blood Sugar Control

Stress and anxiety are intimately linked to blood sugar levels. Elevated stress can lead to poor glucose management, and trouble managing blood sugar can, in turn, heighten stress and anxiety. Understanding how to manage these emotional issues is vital for preserving both physical and mental health.

The Connection Between Stress, Anxiety, and Blood Sugar

Stress triggers the release of hormones such as cortisol and adrenaline, which can cause blood sugar levels to rise. This response is part of the body's fight-or-flight mechanism, which prepares us to respond to perceived dangers. In the short term, this can be advantageous, but persistent stress can lead to protracted periods of increased blood sugar, contributing to insulin resistance and raising the risk of diabetes.

Cortisol and Blood Sugar: Cortisol, known as the stress hormone, promotes gluconeogenesis in the liver, which increases blood sugar levels. Chronic stress leads to sustained high levels of cortisol, which can produce persistently raised blood sugar levels and contribute to insulin resistance.

Adrenaline and Blood Sugar: Adrenaline, another stress hormone, also boosts blood sugar levels by increasing glycogenolysis, the breakdown of glycogen into glucose. This mechanism provides a fast source of energy but can be hazardous when stress is continuous, leading to frequent rises in blood sugar.

Impact on Behavior: Stress and anxiety can also influence behavior, leading to poor eating choices, limited physical activity, and irregular medication adherence. These activities further exacerbate blood sugar control difficulties.

Strategies for Managing Stress and Anxiety

Mindfulness and Meditation: Mindfulness techniques, especially meditation, can dramatically reduce stress levels. These approaches increase present-moment awareness and help individuals manage their reactions to pressures. Research demonstrates that mindfulness can lower cortisol levels and increase overall emotional well-being.

Physical Activity: Regular exercise is a valuable technique for controlling stress. Physical activity raises endorphins, which are normal mood lifters and reduces cortisol levels. Exercise also enhances insulin sensitivity, helping to control blood sugar levels. Activities such as walking, running, yoga, and tai chi can be particularly useful.

Healthy Eating: Maintaining a balanced diet is vital for both blood sugar regulation and stress management. Food's rich in complex carbs, fiber, and healthy fats can stabilize blood sugar levels and minimize spikes and crashes that contribute to stress. Avoiding caffeine and sweets, which can worsen anxiety, is also suggested.

Sleep Hygiene: Adequate sleep is vital for managing stress and maintaining blood sugar control. Poor sleep can increase cortisol levels and insulin resistance. Establishing a regular sleep schedule, providing a tranquil environment, and avoiding stimulants before bed can enhance sleep quality.

Cognitive Behavioral Therapy (CBT): CBT is a highly effective treatment for anxiety and stress. It helps individuals identify and change harmful thought patterns and actions that contribute to stress. CBT can be particularly effective for people with diabetes, helping them build coping mechanisms and enhance their emotional responses to blood sugar management issues.

Support networks: Having a strong support network can ease stress and anxiety. Friends, family, support groups, and mental health experts can provide emotional support, practical counsel, and encouragement. Sharing experiences with others facing similar issues can also alleviate feelings of loneliness.

Managing blood sugar levels is a complicated problem that involves attention to physical, emotional, and psychological health. For women, maintaining normal blood sugar levels is critical for reproductive and sexual health. Understanding the impact of blood sugar on ovarian function, endometrial health, and vaginal health is critical for managing sexual health difficulties. By employing effective measures for glucose control, women can boost their general well-being and improve their sexual health. This includes nutritional changes, regular physical activity, weight management, adherence to medication, and treating psychological and emotional needs. Empowerment via education, support networks, and expert advice can help women negotiate the difficulties of blood sugar management and attain a better, more fulfilled life.

Chapter 4

Managing Blood Sugar for Better Sexual Health

Maintaining normal blood sugar levels is a vital feature of general health, particularly in the context of sexual well-being. Blood sugar, or glucose, is the major energy source for the body's cells, but excessive or insufficient glucose can have far-reaching impacts on physical and mental health, including sexual function. Elevated blood sugar levels can lead to insulin resistance, which can severely damage the vascular and neurological systems, key components in sexual health. Therefore, regulating blood sugar levels by lifestyle adjustments, particularly diet and nutrition, is crucial for boosting sexual health and overall quality of life.

The Importance of a Balanced Diet in Managing Blood Sugar Levels

A balanced diet is the cornerstone of regulating blood sugar levels. It entails consuming a range of foods that give important nutrients while avoiding those that produce rapid spikes and decreases in blood sugar. A balanced diet helps to maintain a constant blood sugar level, which is vital for minimizing the undesirable consequences associated with hyperglycemia (high blood sugar) and hypoglycemia (low blood sugar).

Diet and Nutrition

Diet and nutrition have a crucial role in controlling blood sugar levels. The food we consume is broken down into glucose, which enters the bloodstream and is used by the body for energy. The type and amount of food ingested, the timing of meals, and the balance of macronutrients (carbohydrates, proteins, and fats) all influence blood sugar levels. Therefore, understanding how different foods affect blood sugar is vital for anyone trying to regulate their levels successfully.

Carbohydrates and Blood Sugar

Carbohydrates are the principal source of glucose in the diet. They are found in meals such as bread, rice, pasta, fruits, vegetables, and dairy products. When carbs are ingested, they are broken down into glucose, which enters the bloodstream. The type of carbohydrate—simple or complex—affects how rapidly glucose is released into the bloodstream.

Simple Carbohydrates: These include sugars found in fruits, vegetables, milk, and sweetened foods and drinks. Simple carbs are readily broken down and absorbed, resulting in fast rises in blood sugar levels.

Complex carbs: Found in foods like whole grains, legumes, and starchy vegetables, complex carbs are broken down more slowly, resulting in a steady release of glucose into the bloodstream and a more stable blood sugar level.

Proteins and Fats

Proteins and lipids also have a role in blood sugar regulation. While they do not directly affect blood sugar levels as dramatically as carbohydrates, they influence how rapidly glucose enters the system.

Proteins: Found in meat, fish, eggs, dairy products, lentils, and nuts, proteins can help maintain blood sugar levels by decreasing the absorption of carbohydrates.

Fats: Healthy fats, such as those found in avocados, nuts, seeds, and olive oil, can slow down carbohydrate absorption and can help maintain stable blood sugar levels.

Foods That Help Maintain Stable Blood Sugar Levels

Together with these foods can help to maintain stable blood sugar levels is vital for treating diabetes and boosting overall health. These foods often have a low glycemic index (GI), meaning they promote a slower, more gradual rise in blood sugar levels. Here are some items that can help maintain stable blood sugar levels:

1. Whole Grains

Whole grains, such as brown rice, quinoa, barley, and oats, are good providers of complex carbs and fiber. Unlike processed grains, which have been stripped of their nutrient-rich bran and germ, whole grains retain these components, providing a constant supply of energy and helping to balance blood sugar levels.

Oats: Oats are particularly advantageous due to their high fiber content, specifically beta-glucan, which delays digestion and the absorption of carbs.

Quinoa: Quinoa is a complete protein, including all nine essential amino acids, making it an ideal choice for managing blood sugar levels and providing continuous energy.

2. Vegetables

Non-starchy vegetables, such as leafy greens, broccoli, cauliflower, and peppers, are low in carbohydrates and calories but high in fiber, vitamins, and minerals. These vegetables have a low impact on blood sugar levels and supply critical elements that support overall wellness.

Leafy Greens: Spinach, kale, and Swiss chard are rich in antioxidants, vitamins A, C, and K, and minerals such as magnesium, which help enhance insulin sensitivity.

Broccoli: Broccoli and other cruciferous vegetables contain sulforaphane, a chemical that may help lower blood sugar levels and increase insulin sensitivity.

3. Fruits

While fruits include natural sugars, they also give fiber, vitamins, and antioxidants. Choosing low-GI fruits can help control blood sugar levels.

Berries: Strawberries, blueberries, raspberries, and blackberries are strong in fiber and antioxidants, and have a lower GI compared to other fruits.

Apples: Apples are high in fiber, notably pectin, which can decrease the absorption of sugar and promote gastrointestinal health.

4. Legumes

Beans, lentils, and chickpeas are good sources of plant-based protein, fiber, and complex carbs. They have a low GI and it can assist in maintaining stable blood sugar levels.

Lentils: Lentils are rich in protein and fiber, which can help balance blood sugar and give continuous energy.

Chickpeas: Chickpeas, or garbanzo beans, provide fiber and protein, and their low GI helps in regulating blood sugar levels.

5. Nuts and Seeds

Nuts and seeds contain healthy fats, protein, and fiber, which can help manage blood sugar levels and provide a feeling of fullness.

Almonds: Almonds are rich in monounsaturated fats, fiber, and magnesium, which can increase insulin sensitivity and reduce blood sugar levels.

Chia Seeds: Chia seeds are abundant in fiber, omega-3 fatty acids, and antioxidants, and they develop a gel-like consistency when soaked, which can impede digestion and the absorption of carbs.

6. Dairy and Dairy Alternatives

Low-fat dairy products and fortified dairy alternatives can be part of a balanced diet for regulating blood sugar levels.

Greek Yogurt: Greek yogurt is packed with protein and probiotics, which can help balance blood sugar and improve digestive health.

Almond Milk: Unsweetened almond milk is a low-carbohydrate alternative to dairy milk and can be used in numerous recipes without dramatically altering blood sugar levels.

7. Fish and Lean Meats

Lean proteins, such as fish and chicken, do not immediately alter blood sugar levels and can help maintain a balanced diet.

Fatty Fish: Salmon, mackerel, sardines, and other fatty fish are rich in omega-3 fatty acids, which can reduce inflammation and enhance heart health.

Chicken and Turkey: Skinless chicken and turkey provide lean protein without extra fats or carbohydrates, making them excellent for blood sugar management.

8. Healthy Fats

Including healthy fats into the diet can help manage blood sugar levels and improve general health.

Avocado: Avocado is abundant in monounsaturated fats and fiber, which can help manage blood sugar and create a feeling of satiety.

Olive Oil: Extra virgin olive oil is rich in antioxidants and good fats, which help reduce inflammation and increase insulin sensitivity.

Medications and Treatments

Managing blood sugar levels is critical for patients with diabetes, and drugs play a vital role in maintaining this control. Additionally, various drugs can have diverse implications on sexual health, needing a full understanding of their effects. Alongside pharmacological treatments, non-pharmacological therapies give extra support in managing diabetes and associated consequences.

Overview of Medications for Diabetes and Their Impact on Sexual Health

Diabetes drugs are designed to help regulate blood sugar levels, but their influence on sexual health can vary. Here is a summary of popular diabetic drugs and their potential impacts on sexual function.

1. Metformin

Metformin is a first treatment for type 2 diabetes. It works by lowering glucose synthesis in the liver and enhancing insulin sensitivity. While metformin is generally well-tolerated and does not have a direct detrimental influence on sexual health, it might cause gastrointestinal side effects, which may indirectly decrease libido and sexual performance.

2. Sulfonylureas

Sulfonylureas, such as glipizide and glyburide, stimulate the pancreas to release more insulin. These drugs might lead to hypoglycemia (low blood sugar), which may induce symptoms including weariness, dizziness, and weakness, potentially reducing sexual desire and performance. Additionally, long-term usage of sulfonylureas has been related to weight increase, which can further affect sexual health.

3. DPP-4 Inhibitors

Dipeptidyl peptidase-4 (DPP-4) inhibitors, such as sitagliptin and saxagliptin, act by raising insulin release and reducing glucagon levels in response to meals. These drugs are generally well-tolerated and do not have substantial detrimental effects on sexual health. However, some individuals may develop adverse symptoms like headache and nasopharyngitis, which could indirectly influence sexual well-being.

4. GLP-1 Receptor Agonists

Glucagon-like peptide-1 (GLP-1) receptor agonists, such as exenatide and liraglutide, boost insulin secretion, suppress glucagon release, and slow stomach emptying. These drugs can encourage weight loss, which may positively impact sexual health by enhancing self-esteem and lowering obesity-related sexual dysfunction. However, gastrointestinal side effects, including nausea and vomiting, may impede sexual activity.

5. SGLT2 Inhibitors

Sodium-glucose co-transporter-2 (SGLT2) inhibitors, such as canagliflozin and empagliflozin, act by preventing glucose reabsorption in the kidneys, leading to increased glucose excretion in the urine. These drugs can encourage weight loss and improve blood pressure control, potentially boosting sexual health. However, they may raise the risk of urinary tract infections and vaginal yeast infections, which can significantly impair sexual function and comfort.

6. Insulin Therapy

Insulin therapy is required for persons with type 1 diabetes and some with type 2 diabetes. Insulin helps regulate blood sugar levels by promoting glucose uptake into cells. While insulin therapy alone does not directly impact sexual health, regulating blood sugar levels correctly can improve general health and sexual function. Poor blood sugar control, on the other hand, can lead to consequences such as neuropathy and vascular disorders that significantly influence sexual health.

7. Thiazolidinediones

Thiazolidinediones, such as pioglitazone and rosiglitazone, enhance insulin sensitivity by acting on fat and muscle cells. These drugs might lead to weight gain and fluid retention, which may severely impair sexual health. Additionally, there are concerns regarding cardiovascular hazards connected with thiazolidinediones, which could indirectly influence sexual function.

Non-Pharmacological Treatments and Therapies

In addition to pharmaceuticals, non-pharmacological treatments and therapies play a key role in managing diabetes and its consequences, particularly those linked to sexual health. These treatments focus on lifestyle improvements, psychological assistance, and alternative therapies to increase general well-being.

1. Lifestyle Modifications

Lifestyle modifications are crucial to treating diabetes and improving sexual health. Key lifestyle modifications include:

Dietary Changes

Adopting a balanced diet rich in whole grains, vegetables, fruits, lean meats, and healthy fats helps regulate blood sugar levels and maintain a healthy weight. Avoiding processed foods, sugary beverages, and high carbohydrate consumption is vital. Portion control and mindful eating techniques also help blood sugar regulation.

Physical Activity

Regular exercise raises insulin sensitivity, promotes weight loss, and improves cardiovascular health, all of which contribute to better blood sugar control and sexual health. Aim for at least 150 minutes of moderate-intensity aerobic exercise each week, along with strength training activities two to three times per week.

Smoking Cessation

Smoking negatively influences blood sugar regulation and raises the risk of cardiovascular issues, which can lead to sexual dysfunction. Quitting smoking improves general health and minimizes the risk of diabetes-related problems.

Alcohol Moderation

Excessive alcohol consumption can interfere with blood sugar management and lead to weight gain. Limiting alcohol intake to moderate levels (one drink per day for women and two drinks per day for males) improves blood sugar management and sexual health.

2. Psychological Support

Psychological assistance is vital for persons managing diabetes, as the condition can lead to stress, worry, and depression, which severely influence sexual health. Psychological support can be delivered through:

Counseling and Therapy

Individual or couples counseling can assist address emotional and psychological difficulties related to diabetes and sexual health. Cognitive-behavioral therapy (CBT) and other therapeutic techniques can assist in controlling stress, anxiety, and depression.

Support Groups

Joining support groups for those with diabetes promotes a sense of community and shared experiences. Support groups give emotional support, practical information, and encouragement, helping individuals cope with the problems of managing diabetes and its impact on sexual health.

Stress Management Techniques

Practicing stress management strategies, such as mindfulness meditation, yoga, deep breathing exercises, and progressive muscle relaxation, can help reduce stress and enhance general well-being. Lower stress levels significantly affect blood sugar regulation and sexual health.

3. Alternative Therapies

Several alternative therapies may complement established treatments for diabetes and promote sexual health. These therapies should be used in conjunction with medical guidance and not as a replacement for traditional treatments.

Acupuncture

Acupuncture involves placing tiny needles into particular places on the body to enhance energy flow and facilitate healing. Some research suggests that acupuncture may improve blood sugar control and minimize symptoms of diabetic neuropathy, which can positively enhance sexual health.

Herbal Remedies

Certain plants and supplements, such as fenugreek, bitter melon, and cinnamon, have been examined for their potential to reduce blood sugar levels. However, it is crucial to contact a healthcare expert before utilizing herbal therapies, as they may interfere with diabetes drugs.

Chiropractic Care

Chiropractic care focuses on the alignment of the spine and nervous system to improve overall wellness. Some persons with diabetes find chiropractic adjustments effective for controlling pain and increasing nerve function, which may positively improve sexual health.

Biofeedback

Biofeedback is a technique that teaches humans to manage physiological processes, such as heart rate and muscle tension, through real-time input. Biofeedback may assist persons with diabetes manage stress and improve blood sugar control, contributing to greater sexual health.

Integrating Treatments for Optimal Results

Managing diabetes and its influence on sexual health requires a comprehensive approach that includes both pharmaceutical and non-pharmacological treatments. Collaboration between healthcare providers, including endocrinologists, primary care physicians, nutritionists, psychologists, and alternative medicine practitioners, ensures a holistic and tailored treatment approach.

Regular Monitoring and Adjustments

Regular monitoring of blood sugar levels, HbA1c, blood pressure, and cholesterol levels is vital for assessing the success of therapies and making appropriate modifications. Periodic reviews with healthcare specialists assist optimize medication regimes and lifestyle adjustments.

Personalized Care Plans

Developing tailored care plans that consider individual needs, preferences, and health objectives is critical for optimal diabetes control. Tailored strategies should cover food preferences, physical activity levels, psychological assistance, and alternative therapies.

Education and Empowerment

Education helps individuals with diabetes to take charge of their health. Providing thorough knowledge about diabetes, blood sugar management, medication adherence, and lifestyle changes promotes self-management skills. Empowering individuals to make educated decisions and actively participate in their care improves overall health outcomes.

Effective management of diabetes and its influence on sexual health involves a diverse approach that combines drugs, lifestyle modifications, psychological support, and alternative therapies. Understanding the role of different diabetic drugs and their potential consequences on sexual health is vital for informed decision-making. Integrating non-pharmacological treatments, such as dietary adjustments, regular exercise, stress management, and psychological support, gives a holistic approach to diabetes care. By implementing a thorough and tailored treatment strategy, individuals can achieve improved blood sugar control, boost their sexual health, and improve their overall quality of life.

Chapter 5

Lifestyle Changes and Practical Tips

Managing blood sugar levels efficiently needs extensive lifestyle modifications and practical solutions. These improvements not only improve blood sugar control but also promote overall well-being and quality of life. By adopting healthy habits, individuals with diabetes can control their illness more efficiently and lower the risk of complications.

Healthy Habits for Blood Sugar Management Balanced Diet

A balanced diet is important for maintaining stable blood sugar levels. Here are some nutritional tips to consider:

Emphasize Whole Foods: Incorporate whole grains, fruits, vegetables, lean proteins, and healthy fats into your diet. Whole meals include critical nutrients, fiber, and antioxidants that assist manage blood sugar levels.

Monitor Carbohydrate Intake: Carbohydrates have the most important impact on blood sugar levels. Choose complex carbs, such as whole grains and legumes, which are digested more slowly and have a lower glycemic index. Avoid refined carbohydrates and sugary foods that produce quick blood sugar rises.

Control Portion Sizes: Eating big quantities might contribute to raised blood sugar levels. Use portion control tactics, such as measuring food portions and using smaller dishes, to regulate your intake.

Regular Meal Timing: Consistency in meal timing helps to maintain stable blood sugar levels. Eating at regular intervals, including three main meals and healthy snacks if needed, can reduce blood sugar variations.

Healthy Snacks: Choose snacks that are low in carbohydrates and high in protein or healthy fats, such as nuts, seeds, yogurt, or veggies with hummus. These snacks help keep blood sugar levels constant between meals.

Aerobic Exercise: Engage in aerobic activities such as walking, cycling, swimming, or dancing. Aim for at least 150 minutes of moderate-intensity aerobic exercise per week, distributed across multiple days.

Strength Training: Include strength training exercises, such as lifting weights or utilizing resistance bands, two to three times each week. Strength training develops muscular mass, which helps improve insulin sensitivity.

Flexibility and Balance Exercises: Include exercises like yoga or tai chi to promote flexibility and balance, which can help reduce falls and injuries.

Stay Active Throughout the Day: Reduce sedentary time by incorporating more activity into your daily routine. Take short walks, utilize the stairs, stretch periodically, and engage in activities that involve physical effort.

Stress Management

Chronic stress can negatively affect blood sugar regulation. Implementing stress management practices can help lessen this effect:

Mindfulness and Meditation: Practice mindfulness or meditation to reduce stress and increase relaxation. These approaches can help lower cortisol levels, which can alter blood sugar.

Deep Breathing techniques: Combine deep breathing techniques to relax the nervous system and lessen stress.

Regular Physical Activity: Exercise is a normal stress reducer. Engaging in physical activities you enjoy might help reduce stress levels.

Adequate Sleep: Make sure you get 7-9 hours of quality sleep per night. Poor sleep can impact hormone levels and blood sugar regulation.

Drink Plenty of Water: Make sure to drink at least eight 8-ounce glasses of water every day. Staying hydrated helps maintain normal blood volume and aids in glucose management.

Limit Sugary Drinks: Avoid sugary beverages, such as sodas, sweetened teas, and energy drinks, as they might induce blood sugar rises.

Monitor Caffeine and Alcohol Intake: Limit coffee and alcohol usage, as they can alter blood sugar levels and hydration state.

Establish a Sleep Routine: Go to bed early and wake up at the same time every day, even on weekends. A steady sleep routine helps regulate your body's internal clock.

Create a Relaxing Bedtime Routine: Engage in relaxing activities before bed, such as reading, having a warm bath, or practicing relaxation exercises. Avoid electronics and stimulating activities before bedtime.

Optimize Your Sleep Environment: Ensure your bedroom is cold, dark, and quiet. Invest in a comfy mattress and pillows to increase sleep quality.

Address Sleep Disorders: If you encounter sleep disorders, such as sleep apnea or insomnia, seek medical treatment. Treating these problems can dramatically improve blood sugar control.

Avoid Smoking

Smoking has adverse impacts on blood sugar regulation and overall health. Quitting smoking is one of the finest steps you can take to improve your health and control diabetes:

Seek Support: Utilize smoking cessation programs, support groups, or therapy to help you quit smoking. Nicotine replacement therapy and pharmaceuticals may also be effective.

Understand the Benefits: Recognize that quitting smoking improves blood circulation, and lung function, and reduces the risk of cardiovascular issues connected with diabetes.

Communication with Healthcare Providers

Effective communication with healthcare providers is vital for controlling diabetes and its influence on sexual health. Building a collaborative relationship with your healthcare team ensures that you receive thorough care and support.

Preparing for Appointments

Maximize the efficacy of your healthcare appointments by preparing in advance:

Keep a Health Diary: Maintain a record of your blood sugar levels, medications, symptoms, and any changes in your health. This information gives crucial insights for your healthcare practitioner.

List Your Questions: Prepare a list of questions or concerns to discuss with your healthcare physician.

Prioritize the most essential concerns to ensure they are addressed during the visit.

Bring Your Medications: Bring a list of all your medications, including dosages and any supplements you are taking. This helps your healthcare practitioner analyze your treatment plan and make appropriate adjustments.

Discussing Symptoms and Concerns

Open and honest communication about your symptoms and concerns is vital for optimal diabetes management:

Describe Your Symptoms: Clearly describe any symptoms you are having, including their frequency, duration, and impact on your everyday life. This information helps your healthcare professional detect potential concerns and propose suitable interventions.

Address Sexual Health: If you are experiencing sexual health difficulties, do not hesitate to discuss them with your healthcare physician. Sexual health is a vital element of overall well-being, and your provider can offer information and support.

Discuss Mental Health: Mental health is intimately linked to diabetes treatment. If you are feeling stress, anxiety, or depression, notify your healthcare physician. They can refer you to mental health providers or propose appropriate therapies.

How to discuss sexual health concerns with your doctor

When it comes to sexual health, honest conversation with your doctor is crucial. Here are some stages to steer your conversation:

a. Normalize the Discussion

Start the Conversation: Don't be bashful! Remember that discussing sexual health is a natural component of healthcare. Your doctor is there to help.

Choose the Right Moment: Find a discreet and comfortable environment to share your issues.

b. Specific Concerns

Erectile Dysfunction (ED): If you encounter unreliable erections, communicate this with your doctor. ED is common, and there are medicines available. Your doctor will assess hormone balance and blood flow to the penis1. Pain with Intercourse: If you suffer discomfort during sex, speak it freely. It could be due to several circumstances, including physical concerns or emotional stress.

Vaginal Dryness: Women experiencing vaginal dryness should seek counsel. It can impair sexual pleasure and overall well-being.

Lessened Libido: If your desire for sex has lessened, talk about it. Your doctor can study probable causes and offer strategies.

Importance of Regular Check-ups and Monitoring

Regular check-ups are very important for maintaining general health, including sexual wellness. These visits allow your doctor to uncover any underlying abnormalities early on.

Routine screenings can uncover illnesses including diabetes, heart disease, or hormone imbalances that may influence sexual function2. Mental and Emotional Well-Being

Understand that sexual health is interwoven with mental and emotional components.

Stress and Anxiety: High stress levels can influence sexual desire and performance. Discuss stress management practices with your doctor.

Depression: Depression reduces libido and overall enjoyment. Seek professional help if needed.

Relationship Dynamics: Emotional well-being is directly related to healthy relationships. Address any worries connected to intimacy and communication.

d. Strategies for Coping Holistic Approach: Consider your whole lifestyle. Regular exercise, proper nutrition, and adequate sleep positively improve sexual health.

Communication: Talk openly with your spouse about sexual wants, desires, and boundaries.

Educate Yourself: Learn about sexual health, safe behaviors, and contraception.

Seek Professional Help: If emotional issues impair your sexual health, try therapy or counseling.

Remember, your sexual health matters, and discussing it with your doctor is a proactive step toward general well-being.

Chapter 6

Personal Stories and Case Studies

Personal stories and case studies provide unique insights into the real-life experiences' individuals have with controlling blood sugar levels and their impact on sexual health. These anecdotes demonstrate the challenges, victories, and practical techniques that people use to navigate the intricacies of diabetes and its influence on intimate elements of life. Understanding these stories can offer encouragement, empathy, and practical help for others facing similar challenges.

Real-Life Experiences

The experiences of people managing diabetes are different, reflecting the varied ways in which blood sugar levels might impair sexual health. These anecdotes show the importance of comprehensive diabetes management and the need for open communication with healthcare providers and partners.

Emily's Journey: Managing Diabetes and Restoring Intimacy

Emily, a 45-year-old teacher, was diagnosed with type 2 diabetes five years ago. Initially, she struggled to manage her blood sugar levels, often experiencing large increases after meals. Over time, she found that her sexual drive dropped, and she began to feel vaginal dryness, which made intercourse painful.

Determined to change her position, Emily sought aid from her healthcare practitioner. Her doctor stated that poorly regulated blood sugar levels could compromise vaginal health and sexual performance. Emily was recommended to follow a balanced diet, high in fiber and low in processed sweets, to help regulate her blood sugar levels. She also began a regular workout routine, involving both aerobic activities and strength training.

Emily's doctor gave medicine to assist manage her diabetes more effectively and suggested using a vaginal moisturizer to reduce dryness. Additionally, Emily and her partner attended couples counseling to address the emotional and psychological sides of their relationship.

Over the next year, Emily's blood sugar levels decreased considerably, and she regained her sexual urge. The combination of lifestyle modifications, medicine, and open communication with her spouse led to a more pleasant intimate connection. Emily's story underlines the significance of holistic diabetes care and the good influence it can have on sexual health.

John's Story: Overcoming Erectile Dysfunction

John, a 58-year-old accountant, was diagnosed with type 2 diabetes eight years ago. He maintained his condition relatively well but began having erectile dysfunction (ED) two years following his diagnosis. This issue created tremendous tension and anxiety, impacting his self-esteem and connection with his wife.

John first avoided discussing his ED with his healthcare practitioner out of embarrassment. However, the situation remained, and he decided to seek out treatment. His doctor explained that diabetes could damage blood vessels and neurons, leading to ED. John's blood sugar levels were not effectively controlled, which exacerbated the situation.

To address his ED, John's doctor recommended improving his blood sugar management by dietary changes, more physical exercise, and better adherence to his medication regimen. John also began taking drugs, particularly for ED, which helped restore his sexual function.

John sought help through a local diabetes support group, where he met others facing similar issues. Sharing his experiences and learning from others helped John feel less alienated and more empowered to handle his condition. John's experience shows the significance of obtaining medical care and the positive impacts of community support in managing diabetes-related sexual health difficulties.

Sarah's Experience: Balancing Diabetes and Fertility

Sarah, a 32-year-old marketing executive, was diagnosed with type 1 diabetes at the age of 15. Managing her blood sugar levels had always been a difficulty, but she became more diligent about her health when she and her husband planned to raise a family.

Sarah knew that excessive blood sugar levels could influence fertility and pregnancy outcomes. She worked diligently with her endocrinologist to attain ideal blood sugar management. This included frequent monitoring, modifying her insulin levels, and following a tight meal plan.

Despite her attempts, Sarah endured irregular menstrual periods, which made it difficult to conceive. Her doctor indicated that excessive blood sugar levels could disturb hormonal balance and ovulation. Sarah was referred to a reproductive doctor, who prescribed lifestyle adjustments and followed her attentively.

With the support of her healthcare team, Sarah was able to regulate her blood sugar levels. She integrated stress management strategies, such as yoga and meditation, into her routine to help regulate her periods. After several months of meticulous management, Sarah successfully conceived and had a healthy pregnancy.

Sarah's story highlights the necessity of specialist medical support and lifestyle modifications in treating diabetes and its impact on conception. Her determination and proactive approach were crucial factors in attaining her aim of starting a family.

David's Struggle: Coping with Hypoglycemia and Sexual Health

David, a 50-year-old software engineer, was diagnosed with type 2 diabetes six years ago. He endured frequent periods of hypoglycemia, which left him feeling weak and worried. These incidents generally occurred at night, interrupting his sleep and impairing his overall quality of life.

David found that his sexual desire reduced, and he experienced trouble sustaining an erection. He was concerned about the influence on his relationship with his girlfriend but felt uncomfortable confronting the problem.

During a normal visit to his endocrinologist, David highlighted his issues with hypoglycemia and its influence on his sexual health. His doctor indicated that low blood sugar levels could cause exhaustion, worry, and lower libido. To address the issue, David's doctor modified his medication and recommended a consistent eating schedule to prevent hypoglycemia.

David also started using a continuous glucose monitor (CGM) to better track his blood sugar levels and prevent abrupt reductions. This technology gave real-time data and alarms, enabling him to manage his health more efficiently.

With better blood sugar control and the help of his healthcare team, David's hypoglycemic episodes lessened, and his sexual health improved. Open conversation with his partner and medical specialists was vital in addressing his issues and finding effective answers.

Maria's Transformation: From Depression to Empowerment

Maria, a 38-year-old nurse, was diagnosed with gestational diabetes during her second pregnancy. After having delivery, she continued to suffer from high blood sugar levels and was eventually diagnosed with type 2 diabetes. The diagnosis took a toll on her mental health, leading to melancholy and worry.

Maria's sadness damaged her sexual drive and connection with her husband. She felt overwhelmed by the obligations of controlling her diabetes and caring for her family. Recognizing the need for support, Maria sought counseling from a mental health expert who specialized in chronic illness.

Through therapy, Maria learned to manage her emotions and create healthy cognitive habits. She also joined a diabetes support group, where she bonded with other ladies facing similar issues. The support and encouragement she got helped her feel less alone and more capable of handling her condition.

Maria's healthcare professional worked with her to build a specific diabetes treatment plan, including dietary changes, regular exercise, and medication adjustments.

As Maria's blood sugar levels improved, so did her mood and sexual health.

Maria's path demonstrates the relationship between mental health and diabetes control. Seeking expert therapy and creating a support network were key milestones in her rehabilitation and overall well-being.

Stories from Individuals Managing Blood Sugar Levels and Their Impact on Sexual Health

These individual stories underscore the varied ways in which diabetes can impair sexual health and the significance of comprehensive management techniques. Each individual's journey reflects unique obstacles and answers, offering vital lessons for those experiencing similar circumstances.

Emma and Mark: Strengthening Their Relationship Through Diabetes Management

Emma and Mark, both in their late 40s, were diagnosed with type 2 diabetes within a year of each other. The diagnosis first caused stress and friction in their relationship, as they battled to adapt to new dietary restrictions and lifestyle modifications. Their sexual health also declined, with both having lower desire and intimacy concerns.

Recognizing the need for assistance, Emma and Mark decided to attend diabetes education classes together. These seminars provided students with practical knowledge on controlling their condition and emphasized the necessity of working as a team.

They also sought couples' counseling to address the emotional and psychological impact of diabetes on their relationship. The counseling sessions helped them communicate more effectively and find techniques to assist one another.

Emma and Mark made concerted efforts to enhance their diet and workout habits. They began making nutritious meals together and went for daily walks. These exercises not only helped their blood sugar control but also deepened their friendship.

Through mutual support and shared goals, Emma and Mark made major gains in their diabetes management and sexual health. Their tale shows the value of teamwork and open communication in addressing the problems of diabetes.

Lisa's Path to Empowerment: Overcoming Diabetes-Related Sexual Health Issues

Lisa, a 55-year-old business owner, had been coping with type 2 diabetes for almost a decade. Despite regulating her blood sugar levels pretty effectively, she struggled with vaginal dryness and painful intercourse, which harmed her sexual satisfaction and self-esteem.

Lisa felt ashamed addressing these difficulties with her healthcare practitioner and avoided obtaining help for several years. Eventually, the impact on her quality of life became too significant to ignore, and she determined to address the problem.

Her gynecologist indicated that diabetes could induce changes in vaginal health due to diminished blood flow and hormonal abnormalities. Lisa was administered a vaginal estrogen lotion to reduce dryness and improve her symptoms.

In addition to the medicine, Lisa concentrated on improving her overall diabetes care. She adopted a more balanced diet, increased her physical activity, and employed stress-reduction strategies such as meditation and deep breathing exercises.

Lisa also joined a women's health support group, where she found a secure space to voice her concerns and learn from others' experiences. The support and information she received allowed her to take charge of her sexual health.

Lisa's proactive approach and willingness to seek help led to considerable improvements in her symptoms and overall well-being. Her tale underlines the significance of treating diabetes-related sexual health difficulties and the benefits of obtaining professional care.

Lessons Learned and Practical Advice

The experiences of individuals living with diabetes offer great lessons and practical suggestions for regulating blood sugar levels and enhancing sexual health. These lessons, generated from real-life problems and accomplishments, provide a blueprint for those experiencing similar issues. By evaluating these personal tales, we may discover critical strategies and activities that can lead to better health outcomes and enhanced quality of life.

Importance of Comprehensive Diabetes Management

One of the most essential lessons learned from personal experiences is the significance of thorough diabetes treatment. Effective control of blood sugar levels demands a complex approach that includes food, exercise, medication, and regular monitoring. Individuals like Emily and John, who encountered issues with sexual health due to poorly controlled diabetes, reported considerable improvements when they adopted a holistic management plan. This strategy comprised balanced nutrition, continuous physical activity, and adherence to recommended medications.

Practical guidance for others includes:

Regular Monitoring: Consistently check blood sugar levels to understand how different diets, activities, and medications affect your body. This information can help make required modifications to maintain steady levels.

Balanced Diet: Focus on a diet rich in whole grains, veggies, lean proteins, and healthy fats. Avoid processed foods and sugary snacks that might induce blood sugar increases.

Medication Adherence: Follow your healthcare provider's advice for medication use. Do not skip doses, and discuss any negative effects with your doctor.

Open Communication with Healthcare Providers

Another crucial point is the necessity of open communication with healthcare providers. Many individuals, like David and Lisa, originally hesitated to disclose their sexual health concerns to their doctors. However, when they eventually sought help, they discovered effective treatments and support. Healthcare practitioners can offer valuable assistance, prescribe appropriate medications, and suggest lifestyle modifications that can reduce symptoms and enhance overall well-being.

Practical advice for others includes:

Honesty: Be honest with your healthcare practitioner about any symptoms, especially those relating to sexual health. This transparency enables proper diagnosis and effective therapy.

Ask Questions: Do not hesitate to ask questions regarding your disease, treatment options, and any adverse effects. Understanding your health can empower you to make educated decisions.

Regular Check-Ups: Schedule regular appointments with your healthcare practitioner to check your diabetes treatment and handle any emergent complications promptly.

Emotional and Psychological Support

Personal stories also illustrate the significance of emotional and psychological support in managing diabetes and its influence on sexual health. Many individuals, like Maria, suffered melancholy and anxiety as a result of their diagnosis and its effects on their romantic relationships. Seeking professional treatment from mental health counselors and joining support groups provided them with the tools and encouragement required to cope with these issues.

Partner and Relationship Dynamics

The complexities of relationships play a vital role in treating diabetes and its impact on sexual health. Stories like those of Emma and Mark highlight how teamwork and mutual support may lead to better health results. Couples who work together to control diabetes typically find that their relationships deepen as they negotiate challenges and celebrate victories together.

Practical guidance for others includes:

Open conversation: Maintain open and honest conversation with your spouse about your condition and its effects on your sexual health. This transparency creates understanding and cooperation.

Shared Activities: Engage in activities that promote health and well-being together, such as making healthy meals or exercising. These shared experiences can enhance your friendship and support diabetes management.

Couples Counseling: Consider attending couples counseling if diabetes-related concerns are causing strain in your relationship. A counselor can help you manage these problems and enhance your interpersonal dynamics.

Tailoring Treatment Plans to Individual Needs

Personal anecdotes underscore the need to adapt diabetes treatment programs to individual needs. Each person's experience with diabetes is unique, and what works for one individual may not be helpful for another. Healthcare practitioners must consider each patient's particular circumstances, interests, and lifestyle while designing a management plan.

Practical guidance for others includes:

Personalized Plans: Work with your healthcare practitioner to establish a personalized diabetes treatment plan that meets your requirements and lifestyle. This plan should include food instructions, exercise recommendations, and medication regimes suited to your unique situation.

Flexibility: Be open to altering your treatment strategy as needed. Your demands may alter over time, and your management plan should evolve accordingly.

Self-Advocacy: Advocate for yourself in medical contexts. If you feel that your current treatment plan is not working out, discuss your concerns with your healthcare provider and explore alternate options.

By learning from these personal experiences and adopting the practical counsel they offer, individuals with diabetes can improve their blood sugar control, boost their sexual health, and enjoy satisfying lives. The experiences of others provide useful insights and serve as a source of inspiration and assistance for managing this complex disease.

Chapter 7

Future Directions and Research

Research studying the relationship between blood sugar levels and sexual health is a developing subject matter that shows promise for considerable breakthroughs. As our understanding of the complicated pathways linking diabetes to sexual function deepens, new therapeutic approaches and prevention strategies are expected to emerge. This section discusses the current state of research, potential future paths, and the intriguing role of epigenetics in this domain.

Current Research on Blood Sugar and Sexual Health

Recent research has uncovered numerous routes through which blood sugar levels influence sexual health. Elevated blood sugar, or hyperglycemia, has been associated with several sexual dysfunctions in both men and women, including lower desire, erectile dysfunction, and difficulties in reproductive health. Researchers are concentrating on many important areas to better understand these links and develop effective therapies.

One prominent area for investigation is the influence of persistent hyperglycemia on vascular health. Blood arteries play a critical part in sexual function by giving adequate blood flow to the genital organs. High blood sugar levels can harm the endothelial cells lining the blood arteries, resulting in diminished nitric oxide availability. Nitric oxide is vital for vasodilation and blood flow control. Studies have demonstrated that decreased blood flow due to endothelial dysfunction can result in erectile dysfunction in men and lower genital excitement in women.

Another key concern is the function of inflammation in sexual health. Chronic hyperglycemia causes inflammatory processes that can harm tissues and organs, including those involved in sexual function. Researchers are researching how anti-inflammatory therapies might reduce these effects. For example, research published in the Journal of Sexual Medicine indicated that anti-inflammatory medications could improve erectile function in diabetic men by lowering systemic inflammation.

Hormonal abnormalities generated by elevated blood sugar levels are also a prominent topic of investigation. Diabetes can affect the balance of sex hormones such as testosterone and estrogen, which are necessary for sexual health. Ongoing investigations aim to elucidate the precise processes by which blood sugar regulates hormone production and control. Understanding these systems could lead to specific hormone therapy that restores balance and improves sexual performance in diabetic individuals.

Epigenetic Impact

Epigenetics is an emerging subject that examines how environmental influences and lifestyle decisions can influence gene expression without altering the underlying DNA sequence. Recent research reveals that blood sugar levels can have epigenetic impacts, potentially influencing sexual health throughout generations.

Epigenetic alterations, such as DNA methylation and histone modification, can be altered by metabolic conditions like hyperglycemia. These alterations can alter the expression of genes involved in sexual function, hormone control, and inflammatory responses. For instance, a study in the journal Epigenetics discovered that elevated blood sugar levels could lead to DNA methylation modifications in genes associated with reproductive health, potentially impacting fertility and sexual performance.

Moreover, epigenetic modifications can be inherited, suggesting that the effects of high blood sugar levels might be passed on to future generations. This transgenerational impact raises crucial questions concerning the long-term consequences of poor blood sugar control. Researchers are examining how interventions, such as improved diet and exercise, might reverse negative epigenetic changes and improve sexual health outcomes.

Animal studies have provided solid evidence of the epigenetic impact of blood sugar levels on sexual health. For example, research on rodents has demonstrated that a high-sugar diet can lead to epigenetic alterations that decrease reproductive performance. These discoveries are motivating scientists to study similar processes in humans and create techniques to reduce these consequences through lifestyle modifications and therapeutic therapies.

How Blood Sugar Levels May Influence Future Generations

The impact of blood sugar levels extends beyond acute health issues and can influence the health of future generations through epigenetic pathways. This area of research is gaining prominence as scientists reveal how parental health, particularly related to metabolic problems like diabetes, might affect offspring's risk for numerous diseases, including metabolic and reproductive issues.

Epigenetic Mechanisms

Epigenetics refers to changes in gene expression that do not entail alterations to the underlying DNA sequence. These alterations can be impacted by environmental variables, such as food, stress, and exposure to pollutants. The most researched epigenetic alterations are DNA methylation, histone modification, and non-coding RNA molecules, all of which can control gene activity.

In the setting of blood sugar levels, prolonged hyperglycemia can generate epigenetic alterations that might be passed on to the next generation. For instance, increased blood sugar levels in parents can lead to altered DNA methylation patterns in genes related to metabolic control and inflammation. These alterations can predispose kids to metabolic disorders, including diabetes and obesity.

Influence of Maternal Blood Sugar Levels

Research has demonstrated that maternal blood sugar levels during pregnancy can greatly affect the health of the baby. Gestational diabetes, defined by excessive blood sugar levels throughout pregnancy, is a major issue. It not only raises the chance of problems during pregnancy and delivery but also has long-term health effects for the child.

Studies have revealed that children born to women with gestational diabetes are at a higher risk of acquiring obesity, type 2 diabetes, and cardiovascular problems later in life. This is largely due to epigenetic alterations that occur during fetal development. For example, hyperglycemia can lead to altered DNA methylation in the fetus, altering genes involved in insulin signaling and fat metabolism.

Animal studies provide more evidence of these effects. In rat models, maternal high-fat diets and hyperglycemia have been shown to cause epigenetic modifications in offspring that enhance their vulnerability to metabolic diseases. These findings imply that maintaining normal blood sugar levels during pregnancy is critical for preventing bad health consequences in future generations.

Paternal Contributions

While the majority of the study has focused on maternal impacts, increasing studies highlight the relevance of the father's health in determining offspring's risk of disease. Paternal hyperglycemia can potentially generate epigenetic alterations in sperm that impair the health of the baby.

For instance, elevated blood sugar levels in men have been associated with altered DNA methylation in sperm, which can be passed to the embryo at conception. These epigenetic alterations can affect gene expression patterns in the developing baby, potentially leading to metabolic disorders. Research on rodent models has demonstrated that male mice with diabetes can transmit an increased risk of obesity and insulin resistance to their progeny.

Furthermore, lifestyle factors like as food and physical activity levels in fathers might potentially alter the epigenetic landscape of sperm. Interventions that enhance blood sugar control and overall metabolic health in dads before conception might minimize the chance of passing harmful epigenetic alterations to their children.

The impact of blood sugar levels on future generations through epigenetic inheritance is a fast-emerging area

with substantial implications for public health and
disease prevention. Understanding how hyperglycemia
generates epigenetic alterations that can be passed on to
offspring provides vital insights into the
intergenerational transmission of illness risk.

By concentrating on preconception health, prenatal care,
and intergenerational interventions, we can develop
techniques to reduce the detrimental impacts of elevated
blood sugar levels and promote better health outcomes
for future generations. Continued study in this field will
be critical for identifying specific epigenetic
modifications, understanding their causes, and devising
effective therapies to interrupt the cycle of metabolic
illness transmission.

Chapter 8

Emotional Adjustment and Marital Satisfaction

Living with diabetes can severely damage an individual's mental well-being, which in turn affects their sexual health and overall marital satisfaction. Managing a chronic condition like diabetes demands ongoing awareness and adaptability, which can produce emotional strain and damage interpersonal relationships. Emotional adjustment to diabetes requires coping with the stress and anxiety that come with controlling the disease and comprehending its impact on one's sexual health and marital satisfaction.

Emotional Adjustment to Diabetes

The diagnosis of diabetes typically comes as a shock, bringing about a range of emotions including denial, rage, despair, and eventually acceptance. This emotional rollercoaster can take a toll on an individual's mental health and ability to engage in a happy sexual relationship. The chronic nature of diabetes means that patients must regularly monitor their blood sugar levels, stick to a strict diet, and manage their medication. This continual control can lead to exhaustion and feelings of irritation, which are damaging to emotional and sexual well-being.

Moreover, diabetes can induce physical symptoms such as fatigue, neuropathy, and sexual dysfunction, which can further damage mental wellness. For instance, suffering erectile dysfunction or vaginal dryness can lead to emotions of inadequacy, humiliation, and anxiety about sexual performance. These emotions can produce a cycle of avoidance and decreased sexual engagement, which can undermine marital happiness.

Patients with diabetes need to seek emotional support, whether through counseling, support groups, or therapy. Professional help can provide coping skills to handle the emotional burden of diabetes, helping individuals retain a good outlook and a healthy emotional state, which is crucial for a successful sexual life and marriage connection.

Psychosocial Factors: The Emotional Impact of Diabetes on Sexual Well-being

The psychological components of living with diabetes play a crucial impact in sexual well-being. Psychological stress, anxiety, and despair are widespread among persons managing chronic illnesses, and diabetes is no exception. These mental health difficulties can significantly affect libido and sexual function, generating a complicated interplay between psychological conditions and sexual health.

Psychological Stress and Anxiety

Managing diabetes demands regular attention to dietary choices, blood sugar testing, and medication adherence. This continuous monitoring can lead to chronic stress and anxiety, which are known to impact sexual desire and performance. Stress triggers the release of cortisol, a hormone that can disturb normal hormonal balance and diminish sexual desire. High levels of anxiety can also lead to performance anxiety during sexual engagement, further lowering sexual enjoyment.

Depression

Depression is widespread among patients with diabetes, mainly due to the difficult nature of controlling the disease. Symptoms of depression such as low energy, lack of interest in activities, and negative self-perception can drastically impair libido and sexual satisfaction. Moreover, several drugs for depression can have adverse effects that influence sexual performance, providing a dual difficulty for persons managing both diabetes and depression.

Body Image Issues

Diabetes can lead to weight swings, skin issues, and other physical changes that alter body image. Negative body image can result in low self-esteem and reluctance to engage in sexual activities. Feeling ugly or self-conscious can create a barrier to intimacy, hurting the emotional and physical connection with a partner.

Social Isolation

The necessity for ongoing treatment of diabetes can also contribute to social isolation. Dietary limitations and the need to check blood sugar levels can make social events feel stressful or less pleasurable. This isolation can extend to personal relationships, where the fear of hypoglycemia or other diabetes-related issues might induce patients to forgo sexual engagement, fearing potential embarrassment or discomfort.

Marital Relationships: The Importance of Communication and Emotional Support

In the context of a married relationship, effective communication and emotional support are key components of treating diabetes and sustaining sexual well-being. Diabetes can bring about changes that require both couples to adjust and find new methods to preserve intimacy and connection.

Communication

Open and honest communication is vital for couples dealing with diabetes. Discussing the physical and emotional obstacles offered by the disease can help partners comprehend one another's experiences and sentiments. This mutual understanding can produce a supportive environment where both partners feel appreciated and cared for.

For example, discussing sexual troubles openly can minimize emotions of humiliation and shame, allowing couples to seek solutions jointly. Whether it's seeking medical advice, exploring alternative types of intimacy, or finding strategies to boost sexual pleasure and happiness, communication is crucial to overcoming these problems.

Emotional Support

Emotional support from a partner can considerably relieve the psychological burden of diabetes. Knowing that one is not alone in handling the sickness can give enormous relief and increase mental resilience. Partners can offer assistance by helping with diabetes control activities, providing encouragement, and being empathetic listeners.

Adaptation and Flexibility

Adapting to the changes brought about by diabetes needs flexibility and a willingness to find new methods to retain intimacy. This can require altering the timing or style of sexual activity to meet shifting energy levels and blood sugar levels. Couples may also need to explore various forms of physical intimacy that do not rely only on sexual intercourse but still build closeness and connection.

Strategies for Enhancing Sexual Well-being in Marital Relationships

Managing diabetes successfully can promote sexual well-being and marriage pleasure. Here are some ways that couples can follow to improve their romantic relationships while controlling diabetes:

Lifestyle Modifications

Adopting a healthy lifestyle can enhance both diabetes management and sexual health. Regular physical exercise, a balanced diet, and appropriate sleep are key components of diabetic management that also increase general well-being. Exercise helps increase blood circulation, energy levels, and mood, all of which lead to better sexual health. A balanced diet can assist in maintaining stable blood sugar levels and prevent issues that might compromise sexual performance.

Couples Therapy

Couples therapy can provide a secure space for partners to share their difficulties and establish strategies for preserving intimacy. A therapist can help couples improve communication, manage emotional and sexual difficulties, and deepen their relationship. Therapy can also offer techniques for managing the emotional burden of diabetes, and building a supportive and understanding partnership.

The emotional adjustment to diabetes and its impact on marriage satisfaction and sexual health cannot be stressed. Understanding the psychological elements involved, including the necessity of communication and emotional support, can help couples negotiate the challenges faced by diabetes. By adopting healthy living habits, receiving regular medical treatment, and applying stress management techniques, individuals with diabetes and their partners can boost their mental well-being and maintain a successful sexual relationship. Effective management of diabetes entails not just addressing the physical components of the condition but also promoting strong emotional and relationship health.

Chapter 9

Overcoming Intimacy Challenges in Diabetes Management

Managing diabetes involves multiple physical, emotional, and psychological issues that might hinder intimacy in relationships. Diabetes can induce sexual dysfunction, exhaustion, and emotional anguish, making it difficult to establish a close, personal connection with a partner. However, by knowing these problems and implementing appropriate solutions, couples can overcome obstacles and establish a healthy and intimate relationship despite the presence of diabetes.

Physical Challenges

One of the biggest physical problems that diabetes brings to relationships is sexual dysfunction. In men, this commonly presents as erectile dysfunction (ED), whereas in women, it might include vaginal dryness, decreased libido, and difficulties achieving orgasm. These concerns can result from nerve injury, poor blood circulation, or hormonal abnormalities caused by variable blood sugar levels.

Moreover, the ongoing care of diabetes can lead to exhaustion and a general feeling of malaise, lowering the energy and desire for sexual activity. Hypoglycemia (low blood sugar) can also generate conditions where rapid attention is needed, disturbing moments of intimacy and contributing to anxiety around sexual encounters.

Emotional and Psychological Challenges

Diabetes can have a toll on mental health, leading to stress, anxiety, and sadness. These disorders can further depress sexual desire and present further barriers to connection. Individuals with diabetes could feel self-conscious about their bodies, have anxiety about sexual performance, or worry about their partner's reaction to their condition. This emotional burden can produce a cycle of avoidance and limited closeness.

Strategies for Maintaining Intimacy and Connection in Relationships Affected by Diabetes

Maintaining intimacy in a relationship affected by diabetes demands purposeful effort and open communication. Here are various techniques to assist couples handle these problems and maintain a tight connection:

Education and Understanding

Educating both partners on diabetes and its influence on sexual health is vital. Understanding the physical and emotional repercussions of the disease helps build empathy and avoid misconceptions. Couples can attend diabetes education programs together, read appropriate material, or speak with healthcare specialists to acquire a full awareness of the condition.

Prioritizing Health and Wellness

Maintaining overall health and wellness can greatly improve sexual health and intimacy. Regular physical exercise, a balanced diet, and sufficient sleep are crucial components of diabetic control that also increase energy levels and mood. Exercise promotes blood circulation and can help alleviate symptoms of sexual dysfunction. A diet rich in whole foods, lean proteins, and healthy fats can stabilize blood sugar levels and maintain hormonal balance.

Exploring Alternative Forms of Intimacy

Intimacy is not simply defined by sexual intercourse. Couples might explore various forms of physical and emotional contact that encourage intimacy, such as snuggling, massage, or spending quality time together. Engaging in activities that both partners enjoy and that form emotional relationships can deepen the relationship and provide a sense of intimacy.

Communication Tips for Discussing Intimacy and Sexual Health with Your Partner

Discussing intimacy and sexual health can be tough, but it is crucial for sustaining a healthy relationship. Here are some strategies for fostering these conversations:

Choose the Right Time and Place

Select a comfortable and private environment to discuss intimacy and sexual health. Avoid bringing up sensitive matters during difficult situations or when either spouse is distracted. Finding a peaceful and relaxing environment might make both parties feel more at ease.

Be Honest and Direct

Honesty is vibrant when discussing sexual health and intimacy. Convey your feelings, problems, and desires without laying blame or judgment on your partner. Use "I" sentences to explain your thoughts, such as "I feel worried about my blood sugar levels affecting our intimacy."

Listen Actively

Active listening entails full attention to what your partner is saying without interrupting or formulating your response while they are speaking. Show empathy and understanding, and acknowledge your partner's sentiments. This helps establish a supportive environment where both partners feel heard and valued.

Avoid Blame and Judgment

Approach the talk with sensitivity and avoid blaming or judging your partner. Diabetes and its linked sexual health difficulties are not anyone's fault, and it is crucial to address the topic with a collaborative perspective. Focus on outcome solutions together rather than assigning blame.

Be Patient

These conversations can be unpleasant and may not fix all concerns instantly. Be patient with yourself and your partner as you navigate these. It may take numerous meetings to thoroughly address all concerns and establish appropriate answers.

Seek Professional Guidance

If discussing sexual health and intimacy is overwhelming, try seeking the advice of a therapist or counselor. A professional can facilitate these conversations, provide tools for better communication, and offer assistance in managing the emotional and relational issues of diabetes.

Establish Goals Together

Work together to develop realistic goals for increasing intimacy and managing diabetes. This may involve scheduling regular date nights, trying new types of intimacy, or setting health-related goals such as exercising together. Collaboratively defining goals can enhance the partnership and provide a sense of shared purpose.

Celebrate Progress

Acknowledge and celebrate minor triumphs and progress in managing diabetes and enhancing intimacy. Celebrating victories, no matter how minor, may increase morale and promote positive behaviors and efforts.

Overcoming intimacy issues in diabetes care involves a holistic approach that combines open conversation, practical methods, and emotional support. By recognizing the physical and emotional implications of diabetes on sexual health, couples can work together to discover solutions and maintain a satisfying and intimate relationship. Effective control of diabetes, along with a strong emotional connection, can help couples negotiate the hurdles and have a healthy, intimate partnership.

Chapter 10

Maintaining Healthy Relationships Through Glucose Control

Managing blood sugar levels is a key element of general health for those with diabetes, but it also plays a significant role in sustaining healthy relationships. The physical and mental issues associated with diabetes can hinder intimacy, communication, and the emotional connection between partners. By prioritizing glycemic control, individuals can reduce some of these issues and provide a stronger basis for their relationships. Effective glucose management can help maintain energy levels, improve mood, and lower the risk of problems that could interfere with relationship dynamics.

Physical Health and Intimacy

Stable blood sugar levels can considerably improve physical health, which is vital for maintaining an emotional relationship. When blood sugar levels are well-controlled, individuals are less likely to have physical symptoms that can interfere with relationships, such as exhaustion, neuropathy, or sexual dysfunction. For men, this can mean reducing the likelihood of erectile dysfunction, while for women, it could mean minimizing issues like vaginal dryness or diminished desire.

Consistent glucose regulation helps sustain overall energy levels, making it simpler to engage in physical activities, including sexual activities. When individuals feel physically healthy and active, they are more inclined to initiate and enjoy intimate interactions with their partners.

Emotional Stability and Communication

Blood sugar changes can have a profound impact on emotional stability. High or low blood sugar levels can contribute to anger, anxiety, and mood swings, which can strain communication and emotional relationships in a relationship. By keeping steady glucose levels, individuals can achieve better emotional equilibrium, which is necessary for efficient communication and empathy in a relationship.

When individuals are emotionally stable, they are more suited to tolerate stress and engage in meaningful talks with their partners. This stability enables more constructive and empathic interactions, which are crucial for resolving problems and strengthening emotional ties.

The Importance of Communication and Empathy in Maintaining Healthy Relationships

Open communication and empathy are the cornerstones of any healthy relationship, particularly when one partner is managing a chronic condition like diabetes. The stress and problems associated with diabetes care can be significant, but excellent communication and compassionate support can help reduce these issues and enhance the connection.

Clear, honest communication helps partners to share their wants, worries, and feelings without fear of judgment. It is crucial for both parties to feel heard and understood, which promotes a sense of trust and mutual respect. Regularly addressing how diabetes management is affecting the relationship might help address issues before they become big difficulties.

For instance, discussing the impact of blood sugar levels on mood and energy might assist partners in understanding why certain behaviors or emotions occur. This knowledge can eliminate misunderstandings and animosity, promoting a more helpful and harmonious partnership.

Empathy and Support

Empathy includes understanding and sharing the sentiments of another person. In the context of a relationship affected by diabetes, empathy entails recognizing the daily obstacles and emotional toll that diabetes can have on the afflicted spouse. Providing emotional support, encouragement, and patience can help the person with diabetes feel appreciated and understood.

Empathy also entails being willing to make adjustments in the relationship to fit the demands of the partner with diabetes. This could involve modifications in meal preparation, encouraging healthy lifestyle choices, or being patient during times of emotional or physical distress.

Tips for Prioritizing Intimacy and Connection in Your Relationship

Maintaining closeness and connection in a relationship involves purposeful work, especially when managing a chronic condition like diabetes. Here are some practical strategies for prioritizing intimacy and connection:

Schedule Regular Quality Time

With the busy schedules and demands of daily life, it is crucial to set aside regular time for each other. Scheduling date nights or dedicated time to spend together can help ensure that intimacy and connection remain a priority. This time can be utilized for activities that both partners like, such as going on a stroll, cooking together, or simply talking without distractions.

Focus on Emotional Intimacy

Emotional connection is the basis of a strong relationship. Take the time to participate in deep, meaningful conversations that go beyond surface-level themes. Share your dreams, worries, and aspirations, and actively listen to your partner's thoughts and feelings. Building emotional connections produces a strong relationship that can survive the obstacles of diabetes control.

Be Mindful of Physical Intimacy

Physical closeness is a crucial part of a romantic relationship. However, it is crucial to be cognizant of how diabetes can disrupt physical intimacy and make necessary modifications. For instance, applying lubricants can help ease vaginal dryness in women, and planning intimate times when blood sugar levels are stable can enhance the experience for both parties.

Practice Healthy Lifestyle Habits Together

Engaging in healthy living choices together can deepen the link between partners and promote overall well-being. This could involve making nutritious meals together, exercising as a pair, or finding stress-reducing hobbies that you both like. Supporting each other in maintaining a healthy lifestyle can develop a sense of collaboration and shared goals.

Show Appreciation and Affection

Regularly offering admiration and affection helps reinforce the emotional connection between spouses. Simple actions like expressing thanks, delivering praises, or demonstrating physical love can go a long way in preserving connection. Recognize and congratulate one another's efforts and triumphs, whether great or small.

Address Sexual Health Concerns

If sexual health difficulties emerge due to diabetes, it is crucial to address them openly and get medical treatment. There are treatments and therapies available that can help manage sexual dysfunction and improve sexual health. Consulting with a healthcare expert can provide significant insights and solutions targeted to your requirements.

Manage Stress Together

Chronic stress can negatively affect both diabetes management and interpersonal dynamics. Finding strategies to manage stress together, such as practicing relaxation techniques, indulging in hobbies, or obtaining professional counseling, can help maintain a good emotional balance. Supporting each other during hard times can enhance the connection and develop a sense of unity.

Keep the Spark Alive

Keeping the spark alive in a long-term relationship demands effort and inventiveness. Surprise your lover with kind gestures, schedule surprise outings, or explore new activities together. Keeping the relationship new and unpredictable helps revive the desire and retain a spirit of adventure and enjoyment.

Maintaining successful relationships through glucose control needs a combination of effective diabetes care, open communication, empathy, and conscious attempts to promote intimacy and connection. By understanding the impact of blood sugar levels on physical and mental health, couples can make proactive efforts to address difficulties and enhance their partnership. With the correct methods and support, persons with diabetes can experience rewarding and intimate relationships that withstand the obstacles of managing a chronic condition.

Chapter 11

Technological Advances and Innovations

Technological innovations have substantially impacted the management of diabetes and sexual health, providing new instruments and strategies to monitor and improve both areas of well-being. These developments have made it easier for individuals to monitor their blood sugar levels and treat sexual health concerns, thereby boosting their quality of life.

Continuous Glucose Monitoring (CGM)

Continuous Glucose Monitoring (CGM) technologies have transformed diabetes management. CGM devices continually track glucose levels during the day and night, bringing real-time data and trends. This technology allows users to make more educated decisions about their food, exercise, and medication. By reducing the frequency of finger-prick tests, CGMs offer a less invasive and more thorough approach to monitoring blood sugar.

CGM devices consist of a tiny sensor implanted under the skin, generally on the belly or upper arm. The sensor detects glucose levels in the interstitial fluid and transfers the data to a receiver or smartphone app. This constant feedback helps users spot patterns and respond to changes in glucose levels rapidly, decreasing the risk of hyperglycemia or hypoglycemia.

Insulin Pumps

Insulin pumps give a more flexible and precise means of insulin delivery compared to regular injections. These devices give a continuous infusion of insulin through a catheter implanted under the skin, stimulating the body's natural insulin release. Users can design their insulin pumps to provide basal (background) insulin and bolus doses to cover meals or rectify high blood sugar levels.

Modern insulin pumps commonly interface with CGM systems, forming a closed-loop system, sometimes known as an artificial pancreas. This interface allows the pump to automatically alter insulin supply based on real-time glucose measurements, lowering the strain of diabetes treatment and improving glycemic control.

Smart Pens and Connected Devices

Smart insulin pens and connected devices offer an additional layer of ease and precision in diabetes control. Smart pens can track insulin dosages, document injection timings, and send reminders, helping users prevent missed doses and reduce the risk of dosing errors. These devices generally link with smartphone apps, letting users monitor their insulin usage and communicate data with healthcare providers.

Connected gadgets, such as smart scales and blood pressure monitors, give additional health measures that can inform diabetes care. By integrating these devices into a holistic treatment plan, patients can acquire a greater understanding of how numerous circumstances influence their blood sugar levels and general health.

Mobile Health Apps and Telemedicine

Mobile health apps have become vital tools for managing diabetes and sexual health. These apps offer features such as blood sugar tracking, medication reminders, meal planning, and exercise reporting. Many apps also include educational resources and community support, helping users stay informed and motivated.

Telemedicine has also altered healthcare delivery, making it easier for individuals to get medical advice and support from the comfort of their homes. Virtual consultations with endocrinologists, diabetes educators, and sexual health specialists can provide prompt and individualized care, minimizing the need for in-person visits and increasing patient outcomes.

New Tools and Technologies for Monitoring Blood Sugar and Supporting Sexual Health

Wearable Technology

Wearable technology has moved beyond fitness trackers to include devices specifically tailored for diabetes control and sexual health. Wearable CGM devices, smartwatches with glucose-monitoring capabilities, and wearable patches that distribute medication are just a few examples of how technology is increasing health monitoring.

For sexual health, wearable gadgets that track physiological reactions can provide significant insights. For example, some devices detect heart rate variability, which might suggest stress levels and sexual arousal. By knowing these physiological cues, individuals can better manage their sexual health and address issues such as erectile dysfunction or diminished libido.

Advanced Biosensors

Biosensor technology is continuously improving, giving new ways to monitor health parameters with improved accuracy and convenience. Advanced biosensors can measure glucose levels, hormone variations, and other biomarkers in real-time, offering a comprehensive picture of an individual's health. These sensors can be integrated into wearable devices, smart patches, or even contact lenses, enabling non-invasive and continuous monitoring possibilities.

In the context of sexual health, biosensors can assist in discovering underlying disorders such as hormone imbalances or cardiovascular abnormalities that may influence sexual function. By delivering real-time data, these sensors enable proactive monitoring and rapid interventions.

Artificial Intelligence and Machine Learning

Artificial intelligence (AI) and machine learning (ML) are revolutionizing healthcare by providing predictive analytics and individualized treatment strategies. AI systems can analyze enormous volumes of data from CGM monitors, insulin pumps, and other linked devices to discover patterns and forecast blood sugar variations. This information can help individuals make more educated decisions regarding their diabetes treatment and lower the risk of complications.

In sexual health, AI and ML may analyze data from wearable devices, health apps, and medical records to uncover characteristics that may influence sexual function and enjoyment. Personalized advice based on this study can help individuals address specific concerns and improve their sexual well-being.

Virtual Reality and Augmented Reality

Virtual reality (VR) and augmented reality (AR) are emerging technologies with potential uses in healthcare and sexual health. VR can be utilized for stress reduction, relaxation, and mental health support, which can indirectly enhance diabetes management and sexual health. Guided VR experiences can help individuals practice mindfulness, reduce anxiety, and increase emotional well-being.

AR can deliver real-time information and guidance, increasing diabetic self-management and sexual health education. For example, AR apps can overlay nutritional information on food items or teach proper injection techniques, helping users make informed choices and enhance their health outcomes.

Genomic and Personalized Medicine

Advances in genomics and personalized medicine are paving the way for specific treatments and interventions based on an individual's genetic composition. Genetic testing can uncover predispositions to various disorders, including diabetes and sexual health difficulties. This information can guide tailored treatment programs, lifestyle suggestions, and preventive measures.

For diabetes care, genetic data can improve pharmaceutical selections and dosages, boosting efficacy and decreasing side effects. In sexual health, knowing genetic variables that influence hormone levels, cardiovascular health, or psychological qualities can assist address underlying concerns and enhance treatment outcomes.

Digital Therapeutics

Digital therapies are evidence-based interventions offered through digital platforms, such as smartphone apps or online programs. These therapies can provide behavioral therapy, education, and support for diabetes management and sexual health. Digital therapies offer a convenient and scalable way to give tailored care and enhance health outcomes.

For example, digital therapeutic programs for diabetes control may contain interactive modules on nutrition, exercise, medication adherence, and stress management. These programs can help individuals create healthy behaviors, track their progress, and stay motivated. Similarly, digital treatments for sexual health can give education, therapy, and support for resolving difficulties such as sexual dysfunction, low libido, or relationship concerns.

Technological breakthroughs and innovations are redefining the landscape of diabetes treatment and sexual health, bringing new tools and strategies to improve these areas of well-being. From continuous glucose monitoring and insulin pumps to wearable technologies and digital medicines, these innovations provide more accurate, convenient, and personalized solutions for managing health. By accepting these technologies, individuals can attain improved glycemic management, boost their sexual health, and improve their overall quality of life.

Conclusion

Maintaining good blood sugar levels is crucial for overall well-being. The impact of blood sugar levels extends beyond the management of diabetes; it influences various facets of health, including sexual health, reproductive health, and psychological well-being. This underlines the necessity for comprehensive therapies that involve medicinal interventions, lifestyle adjustments, and psychological support.

Recap of Key Points

In this comprehensive review, we studied several characteristics of how blood sugar levels affect health and well-being. We began by analyzing the physiological components of blood sugar control, such as its impact on sexual health, reproductive organs, and the delicate relationship between blood sugar levels and sexual function in both men and women. We highlighted the significance of maintaining ideal blood sugar levels through nutrition, exercise, and modern medical therapies. We also went into the psychological components, highlighting the emotional and relational implications of diabetes and high blood sugar levels.

Impact on Sexual Health

The association between blood sugar levels and sexual wellness is profound. Higher blood sugar levels can lead to sexual dysfunction in both men and women. For males, elevated blood sugar can induce erectile dysfunction (ED) by harming blood vessels and nerves, limiting blood supply to the penis. It can also impact libido and lead to ejaculation issues. Women may report diminished desire, vaginal dryness, and pain during intercourse due to poor blood sugar regulation. Additionally, hormonal abnormalities induced by diabetes can contribute to irregular menstrual periods and fertility concerns.

Reproductive Health

Reproductive health is substantially influenced by blood sugar levels. In women, elevated blood sugar can disrupt ovarian function, resulting in irregular ovulation and difficulty in embryo implantation due to a damaged endometrial lining. For men, high blood sugar levels can impair sperm quality, decreasing sperm quantity, motility, and morphology. Inflammation and advanced glycation end products (AGEs) play a part in this process, underscoring the significance of regulating blood sugar to protect reproductive health.

Emotional and Psychological Well-being

Blood sugar changes can have a major impact on mood and psychological well-being. Hyperglycemia and hypoglycemia can produce mood fluctuations, irritation, anxiety, and melancholy. These emotional states can further complicate the treatment of diabetes and impair sexual health and relationships. Addressing the psychosocial elements of diabetes is critical for holistic care.

Lifestyle Modifications

Effective blood sugar management entails numerous lifestyle adjustments. A balanced diet high in fiber, lean proteins, healthy fats, and low in refined sugars is vital. Foods that help maintain stable blood sugar levels, such as whole grains, vegetables, and legumes, should be favored. Regular physical activity, including aerobic activities and strength training, can greatly enhance blood sugar control and overall health.

Summary of the Main Takeaways from Each Chapter

Blood Sugar and Sexual Health

The first chapter showed the direct impact of blood sugar levels on sexual health. Elevated blood sugar can lead to erectile dysfunction in men and diminished sexual desire in both men and women. The need to maintain optimal blood sugar levels to prevent these complications was underlined.

Reproductive Health

We studied how blood sugar levels affect reproductive organs, such as the ovaries, endometrium, and sperm. High blood sugar can contribute to irregular ovulation and poor endometrial health in women, while males may have diminished sperm quality. Managing blood sugar levels is vital for sustaining reproductive health.

Psychosocial Factors

The emotional impact of diabetes on sexual well-being and relationships was examined in length. Diabetes can lead to stress, worry, and sadness, which can damage sexual health. Effective communication and emotional support in relationships are key to managing these issues.

Lifestyle Changes and Practical Tips

We went into numerous lifestyle changes and practical techniques for regulating blood sugar levels. This included dietary recommendations, the significance of regular exercise, and the benefits of modern technologies for monitoring blood sugar levels. Embracing these lifestyle adjustments can dramatically improve general health and well-being.

Technological Advances

The role of technological developments in diabetes treatment and sexual health was studied. Innovations such as continuous glucose monitors (CGMs), insulin pumps, and mobile health apps give better control over blood sugar levels and enhance general health.

Final Thoughts on the Importance of Maintaining Healthy Blood Sugar Levels

Maintaining good blood sugar levels is vital for general well-being. Blood sugar levels influence several areas of health, including sexual function, reproductive health, and psychological well-being. Poor blood sugar regulation can lead to major consequences such as erectile dysfunction, diminished libido, reproductive concerns, and emotional disorders.

A comprehensive approach to blood sugar management combines pharmacological therapies, lifestyle adjustments, and psychological support. This includes regular monitoring of blood sugar levels, adopting a balanced diet, engaging in regular physical activity, and utilizing advanced medical tools. Psychological support and appropriate communication in relationships are also vital for managing the emotional burden of diabetes.

Encouragement for Readers

Managing blood sugar levels and increasing sexual health are key parts of overall well-being. It's fair that overcoming these issues might feel daunting at times, but it's crucial to remember that tiny, regular actions can lead to big improvements in both physical and emotional health.

Motivational Message for Managing Blood Sugar and Improving Sexual Health

Managing Blood Sugar:

Managing blood sugar levels is a journey that demands focus and patience. It starts with recognizing the impact of food choices, exercise habits, and stress management on your blood sugar levels. A balanced diet consisting of whole grains, veggies, lean proteins, and healthy fats can help stabilize blood sugar throughout the day. Avoiding sugary beverages and processed foods that produce quick rises in blood sugar is key.

Regular monitoring of blood sugar levels allows you to follow your progress and make educated decisions regarding your health. New technology, like as continuous glucose monitoring (CGMs) and insulin pumps, give vital information and support in managing blood sugar levels properly. Embracing these tools can enable you to take proactive measures toward greater health.

Including physical activity into your routine is another foundation of blood sugar management. Exercise helps your body use insulin more effectively, decreasing blood sugar levels naturally. Aim for a combination of aerobic workouts, like walking or swimming, and strength training to improve muscular strength and overall health.

Improving Sexual Health: Sexual health is a vital element of overall well-being, influenced by both physical and emotional factors. Diabetes and variable blood sugar levels can influence sexual function and desire, but there are techniques to increase sexual health and connection.

Open communication with your healthcare professional and your partner is vital. Discuss any concerns or challenges you may experience relating to sexual health honestly and without hesitation. Your healthcare professional can offer specific guidance and support to help handle these difficulties effectively.

Embrace a healthy lifestyle that supports sexual health. This involves maintaining a balanced diet, remaining physically active, regulating stress levels, and getting enough sleep. These lifestyle variables not only lead to better blood sugar control but also boost overall vitality, which can enhance sexual function and happiness.

Motivational Tips: Set Realistic Goals: Break down your health goals into attainable steps. Celebrate tiny accomplishments along the way to stay motivated.

Stay Informed: Educate yourself on diabetes management, sexual health, and the latest breakthroughs in healthcare. Knowledge empowers you to make informed decisions regarding your health.

Practice Self-Care: Make self-care a priority. Engage in hobbies that bring you joy and relaxation, whether it's reading, spending time outdoors, or practicing mindfulness.

Focus on Progress, Not Perfection: Managing blood sugar levels and increasing sexual health is a long process. Be patient with yourself and accept that setbacks are a natural part of the path.

Final Thoughts: Remember, you can positively impact your health and well-being. By making proactive efforts to regulate your blood sugar levels and prioritize your sexual health, you are investing in a better, more meaningful life. Every action you make towards your health now adds to a brighter and more vibrant future tomorrow.

Embrace the journey of self-care and empowerment. Your health is worth the effort, and with dedication and assistance, you may achieve major changes in both your blood sugar management and sexual health. Here's to a better, happier you!